HOMEMADE AYURVEDA RECIPES COOKBOOK

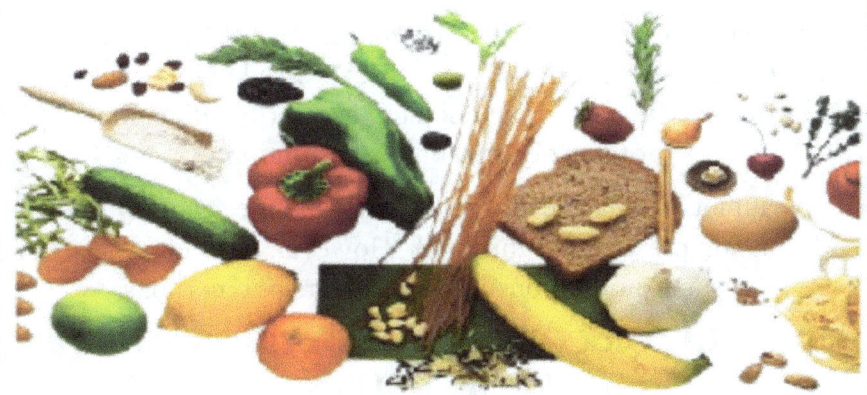

An Essential Ayurvedic Cooking Guide With 55 Delicious Doshas Balancing Meals for Optimal Health and Wellness

Dr. Laura Loeffler

SCAN THIS QR CODE TO GAIN ACCESS TO MORE OF MY BOOKS

Table of Contents

INTRODUCTION

My aunt, who was once an energetic and enthusiastic woman, has been dealing with a variety of health concerns for several years. Her doctor had diagnosed her with a number of diseases, and the medications she was given only provided short respite.

She came upon an Ayurvedic cookbook while visiting a bookshop one day. Ayurveda is an ancient Indian health system that emphasizes the significance of nutrition and lifestyle for total well-being. She was interested and decided to give it a shot.

She discovered a comprehensive approach to wellness that went beyond diet as she dug more into Ayurvedic ideas. She discovered the significance of balancing her doshas, the three primary energy kinds in the body, as well as how to select foods and lifestyle choices that would benefit her specific constitution.

She began adopting Ayurvedic concepts into her daily practice with renewed zeal. She began making healthful Ayurvedic meals from the cookbook, and she also began practicing yoga and meditation on a daily basis.

Within a few months, she noticed a significant improvement in her health. Her energy levels skyrocketed, her stomach troubles vanished, and her general sense of well-being greatly improved. She was astounded by Ayurveda's transformational power and the influence it had on her life.

The plant-centric, whole-food component of the Ayurvedic diet benefited not just her physical health but also her emotional well-being. Her Ayurvedic experience underscored the ancient practice's holistic approach, emphasizing the balance between individual energy patterns and universal components to promote total health and vitality.

My aunt became an advocate for Ayurvedic life after being inspired by her personal path. She passed on her knowledge and experience to others, urging them to investigate the healing possibilities of this ancient wisdom. She is now a live example of the power of Ayurveda, leading a healthy, balanced, and meaningful life.

Purpose of the Book

Welcome to the "Homemade Ayurveda Recipes Cookbook," a journey into the rich and ancient heritage of Ayurveda, where food is transformed into a means of achieving overall well-being. This book was written with the goal of educating you to embrace the healing possibilities of your kitchen and make educated decisions that align with Ayurvedic principles.

The need for sustainable and preventative methods has never been higher in today's fast-paced society, where health issues abound. This cookbook is more than simply a collection of recipes; it is an invitation to go on a transforming culinary experience based on Ayurvedic teachings. We celebrate the concept that, when addressed wisely, food can be a potent source of healing as well as nourishment.

My goal is twofold: first, to demystify Ayurveda and make its principles accessible to anyone, regardless of prior knowledge; and second, to promote the practice of Ayurveda. Second, to assist you in developing wholesome meals that are tailored to your individual constitution, fostering balance and vigor. Imagine a kitchen filled with the fragrances of therapeutic spices and the brilliant colors of nourishing ingredients as you read through these pages, setting the stage for a better and more peaceful existence.

Understanding Ayurveda: A Brief Overview

To truly comprehend the recipes that follow, let's first learn about Ayurveda, a traditional health system that began in ancient India over 5,000 years ago. Ayurveda, which means "knowledge of life," is a holistic health method that strives to balance the mind, body, and spirit.

At its foundation, Ayurveda respects each individual's unique constitution, known as their dosha. Vata, Pitta, and Kapha are the three basic doshas, each representing a mixture of the five elements (earth, water, fire, air, and ether). Understanding your dominant dosha is essential for balancing your lifestyle, including your food.

Vata, which is related to air and ether, regulates mobility and is associated with traits such as dryness and lightness. Pitta, which is associated with fire and water, controls digestion and is distinguished by heat and intensity. Kapha, which is anchored in earth and water, regulates construction and demonstrates weight and solidity.

Ayurveda also recognizes the doshas' dynamic interplay inside us and their effect on our mental, emotional, and physical states. Imbalances in the doshas can cause a variety of health problems, and Ayurveda provides tailored techniques for restoring balance.

In this quick review, we lay the groundwork for a more in-depth study of Ayurveda, preparing you to go on a holistic gastronomic adventure. Keep in mind the knowledge of Ayurveda and how it connects with your individual constitution as you explore the recipes ahead for maximum well-being.

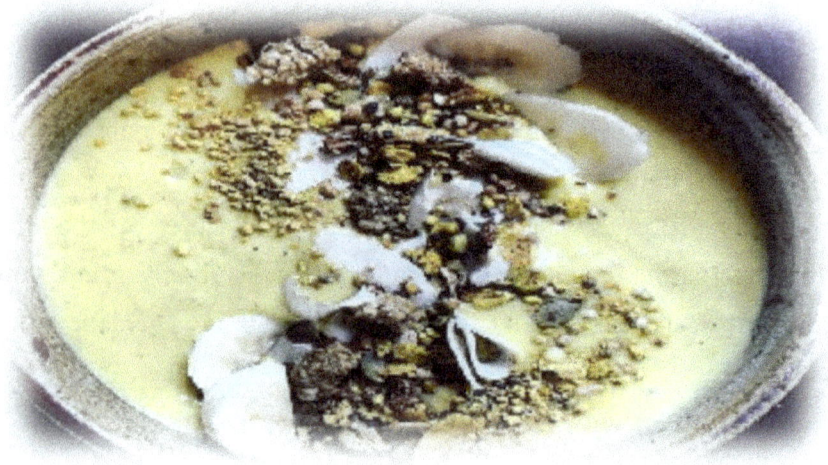

How food impacts health in Ayurveda

Now that we've covered the essentials, let's look into the significant relationship between food and health in the Ayurvedic setting. Food is seen as a powerful kind of medicine in Ayurveda, capable of either fostering or upsetting the delicate balance of the doshas.

Every bite we take has an effect on our digestive balance, affecting our energy levels, digestion, and general well-being. Ayurvedic food classification is based on taste (rasa), quality (guna), and post-digestive effects (vipaka). Sweet, sour, salty, pungent, bitter, and astringent are the six flavors that play an important part in constructing a balanced meal that satisfies all the doshas.

To counteract its dry and light traits, Vata, for example, benefits from warm, nutritious meals with sweet, sour, and salty flavors. To counter its fiery character, Pitta thrives on cooling, hydrating meals with sweet, bitter, and astringent flavors. To combat its heaviness, Kapha prefers warm, light, and spicy meals with pungent, bitter, and astringent flavors.

Food properties, such as whether it is heavy or light, hot or cold, wet or dry, all have an effect on the doshas. Understanding these characteristics enables us to make educated decisions, such as choosing meals that complement our specific constitution and correcting imbalances.

Furthermore, Ayurveda emphasizes the value of mindful eating habits, such as paying attention to food seasonality, eating in a peaceful atmosphere, and being present throughout meals. This holistic approach encompasses the full experience of sustaining oneself, not just the foods on our plate.

In the following chapters, you'll find recipes meant to tap into the medicinal potential of Ayurvedic principles. By adopting these dishes into your everyday life, you will go on a culinary adventure that will not only satisfy your taste buds but will also encourage balance, energy, and a deeper connection with Ayurvedic wisdom. Prepare to enjoy the taste of well-being!

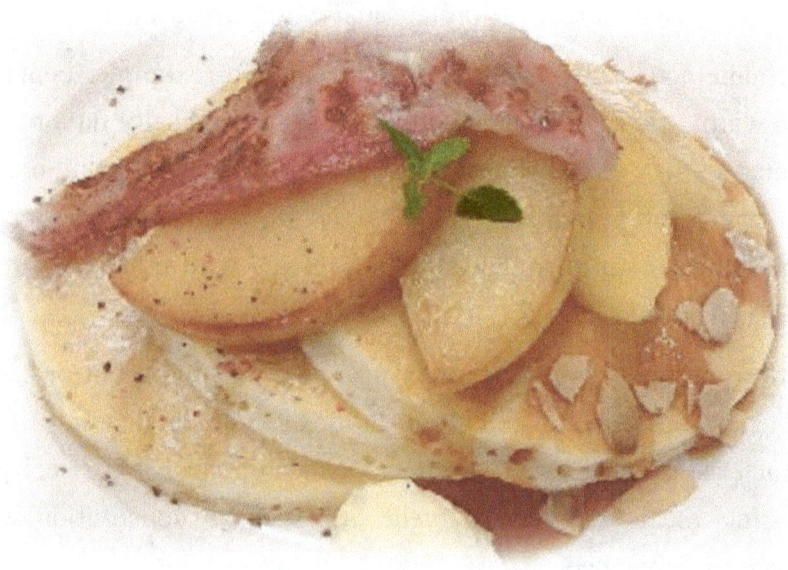

CHAPTER 1

The Principles of Ayurveda

Ayurveda is based on a deep awareness of the interconnection of all elements of our being; physical, mental, and spiritual. Ayurvedic principles are based on the notion that each individual is a unique blend of the five elements: earth, water, fire, air, and ether. These components combine to generate three basic energies known as doshas: vata, pitta, and kapha.

Understanding Doshas: Your Personality

To understand Ayurvedic principles, one must first understand the notion of doshas, which are the basic forces that regulate our physiological and psychological activities. Everyone has a unique blend of these doshas, which determines everything from our physical appearance to our mental predispositions.

1. **Vata:** The elements of air and ether govern Vata, which embodies attributes of mobility, lightness, and variety. People with a strong Vata constitution are creative, lively, and quick to think. An imbalance in Vata, on the other hand, might appear as anxiety, restlessness, and digestive difficulties.

2. **Pitta** regulates metabolism, digestion, and transformation and is associated with the elements fire and water. Pitta-dominant people are known for their passion, acute intellect, and powerful digestion. Pitta imbalance can cause irritation, inflammation, and digestive problems.

3. **Kapha:** Rooted in the soil and water elements, Kapha represents stability, structure, and nutrition. Those with a Kapha constitution have a strong and consistent presence, both physically and emotionally. Kapha imbalances can cause fatigue, weight gain, and respiratory problems.

Recognizing the dosha or combination of doshas that is most dominant in your composition is the first step in understanding your unique constitution. In Ayurveda, this awareness acts as a guiding principle, informing lifestyle decisions, food preferences, and general well-being practices.

The Importance of Dosha Balancing

Ayurveda emphasizes the necessity of maintaining a harmonic balance of the doshas in the delicate dance of life. Imbalances can arise as a result of a variety of variables, such as nutrition, lifestyle, stress, and environmental effects. When a dosha is inflamed or decreased, it can cause a chain reaction of physical and mental health problems.

1. **Balancing Vata:** Incorporating warm, nutritious foods and creating regular routines are critical for people with excess Vata. Warm soups and stews, as well as grounding exercises like yoga and meditation, can help calm excess vata energy.

2. **Pitta balance:** People who have an excess of Pitta benefit from cooling and hydrating meals. Pitta can be balanced by adopting a quiet and peaceful lifestyle, avoiding spicy or hot meals, and engaging in activities that promote tranquility.

3. **Balancing Kapha:** Focus on exciting and revitalizing techniques to balance Kapha. Light, spicy meals, regular

exercise, and a dynamic daily routine can all help counteract the immobility that comes with too much Kapha.

Ayurveda emphasizes that balance is a dynamic equilibrium that requires constant observation and correction. It encourages people to become more aware of their bodies', emotions', and surroundings and to make deliberate decisions to restore and maintain balance.

Ayurvedic Lifestyle Practices

B eyond dietary considerations, Ayurveda encompasses a holistic approach to life that extends to various lifestyle practices. These practices aim to align individuals with the natural rhythms of the universe, fostering a sense of well-being and harmony.

1. **Daily Routines (Dinacharya):** Ayurveda emphasizes the importance of daily routines to synchronize our internal biological clock with the external environment. This includes practices such as waking up early, tongue scraping, oil pulling, and self-massage with warm oils tailored to one's dosha.

2. **Seasonal Adjustments (Ritucharya):** Recognizing that each season has a unique influence on the doshas, Ayurveda suggests seasonal adjustments to maintain balance. For example, cooling foods and practices are recommended in the heat of summer, while warming and grounding approaches are favored during the colder months.

3. **Yoga and Exercise:** Physical activity is considered crucial in Ayurveda for maintaining optimal health. Tailored to individual

doshas, yoga and exercise practices help improve circulation, enhance digestion, and promote overall vitality.

4. **Meditation and mindfulness:** Ayurveda places a strong emphasis on mental well-being. Practices such as meditation, mindfulness, and pranayama (breath control) are recommended to calm the mind, reduce stress, and promote emotional balance.

5. **Connecting with Nature:** Ayurveda acknowledges the healing power of nature. Spending time outdoors, practicing grounding techniques, and cultivating an appreciation for the natural world contribute to overall well-being.

6. **Social and Emotional Health:** Healthy relationships and emotional well-being are integral components of Ayurvedic living. Nurturing positive connections, practicing gratitude, and engaging in activities that bring joy contribute to emotional balance.

In essence, Ayurvedic lifestyle practices are a roadmap for individuals to navigate the complexities of modern life while staying true to their unique constitution. By integrating these practices into daily life, individuals can cultivate resilience, adaptability, and a deep sense of holistic well-being.

As we journey through the principles of Ayurveda, from understanding the doshas to embracing lifestyle practices, the overarching theme is one of self-awareness and harmony. Ayurveda invites us to embark on a journey of self-discovery, recognizing the interconnectedness of our body, mind, and spirit. In the chapters that follow, we'll delve deeper into the practical application of these principles through the art of Ayurvedic cooking, guiding you towards a path of balance, vitality, and lasting well-being.

CHAPTER 2

Key Ingredients for Ayurvedic Cooking

Embarking on a journey into Ayurvedic cooking involves not just recipes but a thoughtful curation of your pantry. Ayurveda, the ancient system of medicine from India, places a strong emphasis on the connection between food and health. The Ayurvedic pantry is a treasure trove of whole foods, spices, and oils that support balance and well-being. Let's delve into the essential components that form the backbone of Ayurvedic culinary exploration.

1. **Whole grains:** Whole grains serve as the cornerstone of Ayurvedic cooking, providing a sustained source of energy and vital nutrients. Basmati rice, quinoa, barley, and millet are staples that form the basis of nourishing meals. Opt for whole, unprocessed grains to maximize their nutritional content and support digestive health.

2. **Legumes:** Rich in plant-based protein and fiber, legumes are a crucial element in Ayurvedic cuisine. Lentils, mung beans, chickpeas, and black beans are versatile options that can be used in soups, stews, and salads. Soaking legumes before cooking aids in their digestibility and enhances nutrient absorption.

3. **Seeds and nuts:** Seeds and nuts add texture, flavor, and a nutritional boost to Ayurvedic dishes. Incorporate sesame seeds, sunflower seeds, chia seeds, almonds, and walnuts into

your pantry. These nutrient-dense options contribute essential fats, proteins, and micronutrients to your meals.

4. Spice Rack Essentials: The spice rack is the heartbeat of Ayurvedic cooking, infusing dishes with flavor and therapeutic benefits. A well-stocked spice rack includes:

✓ **Turmeric:** Known for its anti-inflammatory properties, turmeric adds a warm, golden hue to dishes.

✓ **Cumin:** With a slightly nutty flavor, cumin aids digestion and is often used in spice blends.

✓ **Coriander:** Both the seeds and the fresh leaves (cilantro) are utilized, offering a citrusy, aromatic quality.

✓ **Fennel Seeds:** A digestive aid, fennel seeds add a sweet and licorice-like flavor to dishes.

✓ **Mustard Seeds:** These tiny seeds bring a pungent kick to dishes and stimulate digestion.

✓ **Cardamom:** A fragrant spice with a hint of citrus, cardamom is used in both sweet and savory recipes.

✓ **Cinnamon:** Balancing sweetness and warmth, cinnamon is a versatile spice in Ayurvedic cooking.

✓ **Ginger and garlic:** These aromatic roots are essential for flavor and digestive benefits.

✓ **Asafoetida (Hing):** Used in minimal amounts, asafoetida enhances digestion and reduces flatulence.

The Role of Ghee and Healthy Oils

G hee, or clarified butter, holds a revered place in Ayurvedic cooking. Known for its rich, nutty flavor and digestive benefits, ghee is suitable for all three doshas. It has a high smoke point, making it ideal for sautéing and frying. Additionally, ghee is believed to carry the medicinal properties of herbs and spices when used in cooking.

Healthy oils, such as sesame oil, coconut oil, and olive oil, are also valued in Ayurveda. Each oil has unique properties, and their selection depends on individual doshas and specific cooking requirements. Sesame oil is often used for its warming nature, while coconut oil adds a cooling element.

Sweeteners and Flours in Ayurveda

Ayurveda encourages the use of natural sweeteners and wholesome flours to enhance the nutritional value of dishes. Consider incorporating the following:

1. **Sweeteners:** Opt for honey, jaggery, or maple syrup instead of refined sugars. These sweeteners provide additional minerals and have varying effects on the doshas.

2. **Flours:** Whole-grain flours, such as whole wheat, barley, and millet flour, offer a nutrient-dense alternative to refined flours. Explore gluten-free options like rice flour and chickpea flour for diversity in your recipes.

The Six Tastes in Ayurveda

A yurveda recognizes six tastes, each associated with specific elements and doshas. Integrating these tastes into your meals promotes balance and satisfies the diverse needs of the body. The six tastes are:

1. **Sweet (Madhura):** The sweet taste is grounding, nourishing, and calming. It is related with the elements of earth and water. Foods like fruits, grains, and natural sweeteners provide a sweet taste, offering comfort and stability.

2. **Sour (Amla):** The sour flavor is associated with the elements fire and earth. It stimulates digestion and kindles agni (digestive fire). Sour foods include citrus fruits, tomatoes, and fermented foods like yogurt and vinegar.

3. **Salty (Lavana):** A salty taste corresponds to water and fire elements. It enhances taste perception, stimulates digestion, and aids in the elimination of waste. Sea salt, rock salt, and naturally salty foods like seaweed contribute to this taste.

4. **Pungent (Katu):** The pungent taste is associated with fire and air elements. It stimulates digestion, promotes circulation, and has a heating effect. Pungent foods include spices like chili peppers, black pepper, garlic, and ginger.

5. **Bitter (Tikta):** Bitter taste is linked to the air and ether elements. It has a cooling and detoxifying effect on the body. Bitter foods include leafy greens, turmeric, fenugreek, and bitter melon.

6. **Astringent (Kashaya):** An astringent taste is associated with the air and earth elements. It has a drying and toning effect, helping to balance excessive moisture in the body. Astringent foods include legumes, certain fruits like pomegranate, and green tea.

Balancing Tastes for Optimal Health

A yurveda emphasizes the importance of incorporating all six tastes into each meal to create a well-rounded and satisfying eating experience. Balancing tastes ensures that all the doshas are addressed, promoting optimal health and preventing imbalances. Consider the following guidelines:

1. **Vata-Pacifying Tastes:** Sweet, sour, and salty tastes help balance Vata's dry and light qualities. Emphasize nourishing, warm, and moist foods.

2. **Pitta-Pacifying Tastes:** Sweet, bitter, and astringent tastes are cooling and soothing for Pitta. Opt for foods that balance heat and acidity, avoiding excessive pungent, sour, and salty tastes.

3. **Kapha-Pacifying Tastes:** Bitter, pungent, and astringent tastes help counter Kapha's heavy and cold qualities. Focus on foods that are light, warm, and exciting.

Creating Harmony with a Variety of Tastes

A yurveda encourages a varied and seasonal diet that incorporates all six tastes to maintain balance. Each taste contributes specific qualities to a meal, and their combination determines the overall effect on the doshas. Here are some tips for creating harmony with a variety of tastes:

1. **Diverse Meals:** Aim for a diverse array of tastes in each meal, incorporating a mix of sweet, sour, salty, pungent, bitter, and astringent flavors.

2. **Seasonal Adjustments:** Adjust your diet according to the seasons to align with nature's cycles. In colder months, favor warm and grounding tastes, while cooler months may call for lighter and more cooling flavors.

3. **Mindful Pairing:** Be mindful of taste combinations to enhance the overall dining experience. For example, balancing the heat of pungent spices with the sweetness of fruits can create a harmonious blend.

4. **Personalized Approach:** Consider your individual constitution and any current imbalances when planning meals. Tailor the tastes to address specific needs and promote overall well-being.

By understanding the six tastes and their impact on the doshas, you gain a powerful tool for creating meals that support balance, satisfaction, and optimal health. As we continue our exploration of Ayurvedic cooking, these principles will guide the creation of flavorful and nourishing dishes that resonate with the wisdom of this ancient tradition.

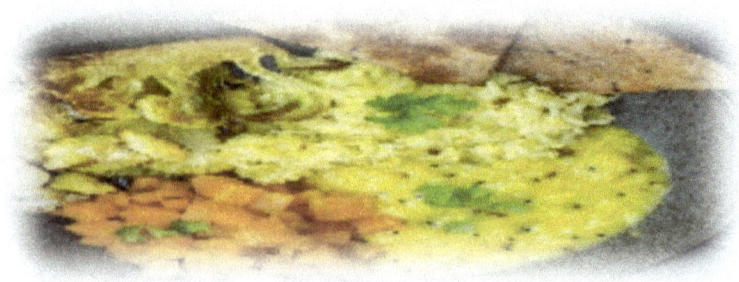

CHAPTER 3
BREAKFAST DELIGHTS
Energizing Morning Recipes
1. Raw Soaked Oatmeal with Pumpkin Seeds and Apricots

Ingredients:

✓ 1 cup rolled oats

✓ 2 cups almond milk (or any preferred milk)

✓ 2 tablespoons chia seeds

✓ 2 tablespoons pumpkin seeds

✓ 4-5 dried apricots, chopped

✓ 1 tablespoon honey or maple syrup

✓ 1/2 teaspoon ground cinnamon

✓ A pinch of salt

✓ Fresh fruits (such as berries or sliced banana) for garnish (optional)

Preparation:

1. In a bowl, combine rolled oats and almond milk.

2. Add chia seeds, stir well, and let the mixture soak for at least 30 minutes or refrigerate overnight for a convenient morning preparation.

3. After soaking, stir in pumpkin seeds, chopped dried apricots, honey or maple syrup, ground cinnamon, and a pinch of salt.

4. To achieve a uniform distribution of components, carefully mix

5. Garnish with fresh fruits like berries or sliced banana if desired.

6. Serve the raw soaked oatmeal chilled, straight from the refrigerator.

7. Customize with additional toppings like nuts, seeds, or a dollop of yogurt if desired.

Total Nutritional Value (Approximate): Calories: 563, Total Fat: 24.4g, Carbohydrates: 76g, Dietary Fiber: 17.5g, Protein: 17g.

Preparation Time: 5 minutes (excluding soaking time)

Soaking Time: Minimum 30 minutes, or overnight for added convenience.

This raw soaked oatmeal is a delightful and nourishing breakfast option that aligns with Ayurvedic principles. It incorporates a balance of tastes, supports digestion, and provides a mix of essential nutrients to kickstart your day with vitality and wellness. Adjust ingredient quantities to suit your preferences and dosha constitution, and enjoy this wholesome and satisfying breakfast.

2. Cream of Rice Soup (Congee)

Ingredients:

✓ 1/2 cup white Basmati rice

✓ 4 cups water

✓ 1 tablespoon ghee

✓ 1/2 teaspoon cumin seeds

✓ 1/2 teaspoon mustard seeds

✓ 1/2 teaspoon turmeric powder

✓ 1/2 teaspoon ginger, grated

✓ 1/2 cup carrots, finely chopped

✓ 1/2 cup zucchini, finely chopped

✓ 4 cups vegetable broth

✓ 1/2 cup coconut milk

✓ Salt to taste

✓ Fresh cilantro for garnish (optional)

✓ Squeeze of fresh lemon juice (optional)

Preparation:

1. Use cold water to rinse the Basmati rice until it becomes clean.

2. Soak the rice in water for 15-20 minutes to enhance digestibility.

3. In a pot, combine soaked rice and 4 cups of water.

4. Bring to a boil, then turn down to a lower heat.

5. Cook until the rice is soft and begins to break down, stirring occasionally (approximately 20-30 minutes).

6. Heat the ghee in a separate pan over average heat.

7. Add cumin seeds and mustard seeds. Once they start to splutter, add turmeric powder and grated ginger. Sauté for a minute until aromatic.

8. Add finely chopped carrots and zucchini to the spice base.

9. Cook for 3-5 minutes until the vegetables are slightly tender.

10. Once the rice is cooked, add the vegetable mixture to the rice pot.

11. Pour in vegetable broth and coconut milk. Stir well to combine.

12. Simmer the congee over low heat for an additional 15-20 minutes, allowing the flavors to meld and the soup to thicken.

13. Season with salt to taste.

14. If preferred, garnish with fresh cilantro and a squeeze of fresh lemon juice.

Total Nutritional Value (Approximate Per Serving): Calories: 364, Total Fat: 25.2g, Carbohydrates: 33.9g, Dietary Fiber: 3.8g, Protein: 4.4g.

9. Cooking Time:

✓ **Preparation Time:** 15 minutes (excluding rice soaking time).

✓ **Cooking Time:** 50-60 minutes (including rice cooking and simmering).

This Cream of Rice Soup (Congee) is a comforting and nutritious breakfast option. It aligns with Ayurvedic principles by incorporating warming spices, nourishing vegetables, and easily digestible rice. Adjust ingredient quantities based on personal preferences and dosha considerations for a wholesome start to your day

3. Savory Corn Pancakes

Ingredients:

✓ 1 cup cornmeal

✓ 1/2 cup whole wheat flour

✓ 1/2 cup plain yogurt

✓ 1/2 cup water

✓ 1 cup fresh or frozen corn kernels

✓ 1/4 cup finely chopped red bell pepper

✓ 1/4 cup finely chopped green onions

✓ 1 teaspoon grated ginger

- ✓ 1/2 teaspoon cumin powder
- ✓ 1/2 teaspoon coriander powder
- ✓ 1/4 teaspoon turmeric powder
- ✓ 1/4 teaspoon black pepper
- ✓ 1/2 teaspoon baking soda
- ✓ Salt to taste
- ✓ Ghee or oil for cooking

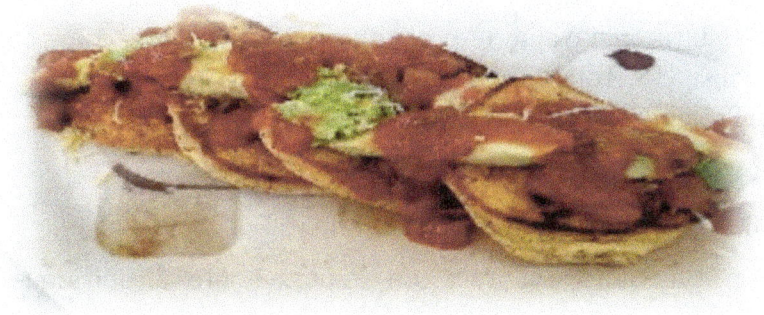

Preparation:

1. In a mixing bowl, combine cornmeal, whole wheat flour, plain yogurt, and water to make a smooth batter. Let it rest for 15 minutes.

2. Add corn kernels, finely chopped red bell pepper, green onions, grated ginger, cumin powder, coriander powder, turmeric powder, black pepper, baking soda, and salt to the batter.

3. Mix well to incorporate the vegetables and spices.

4. If the batter is too thick, add a little more water to achieve a pouring consistency.

5. Preheat a nonstick skillet or griddle over average heat.

6. Add a teaspoon of ghee or oil.

7. Pour a ladle of batter onto the hot pan to form a pancake. Spread it gently to the desired thickness.

8. Cook until the edges start to brown and bubbles appear on the surface.

9. Cook the opposite side of the pancake until golden brown.

10. Repeat with the remaining batter, using extra ghee or oil as necessary.

Total Nutritional Value (Approximate Per Serving - 2 Pancakes): Calories: 818, Total Fat: 8.8g, Carbohydrates: 165g, Dietary Fiber: 20g, Protein: 26.5g.

Preparation Time: 20 minutes

Cooking Time: 15 minutes

These Ayurvedic Savory Corn Pancakes are a nutritious and wholesome breakfast option, combining the goodness of cornmeal, whole wheat flour, and a variety of vegetables and spices. Enjoy them with your favorite chutney or yogurt for a satisfying start to your day. Adjust ingredients based on your dosha or personal preferences.

4 Apple Sauce with Ginger & Ghee

Ingredients:

✓ 4 medium-sized apples, peeled, cored, and diced

✓ 1 tablespoon ghee

✓ 1 teaspoon fresh ginger, grated

✓ 1/2 teaspoon ground cinnamon

✓ 1/4 teaspoon ground cardamom

✓ 1-2 tablespoons honey or maple syrup (modify to flavor)

✓ 1/4 cup water

✓ Chopped nuts (almonds or walnuts) for garnish (optional)

Preparation:

1. Peel, core, and dice the apples.

2. Melt the ghee in a pot over average heat.

3. Add diced apples and sauté for 3-5 minutes until they begin to soften.

4. Stir in grated ginger, ground cinnamon, and ground cardamom.

5. Continue to sauté for an additional 2-3 minutes to infuse the flavors.

6. Pour 1/4 cup of water into the saucepan to help the apples cook and create a sauce.

7. Cover the pan and simmer for 10-15 minutes or until the apples are tender.

8. Using a fork or potato masher, mash the softened apples to achieve the desired consistency.

9. Add honey or maple syrup to sweeten the applesauce.

10. Sweetness can be adjusted to your preference.

11. Optional: Garnish with chopped nuts (almonds or walnuts) for added texture and nutritional value.

Total Nutritional Value (Approximate Per Serving): Calories: 518-542, Total Fat: 17.72-18.72g, Carbohydrates: 113.47-113.97g, Dietary Fiber: 14.1g, Protein: 3.16-3.16g.

Preparation Time: 10 minutes

Cooking Time: 20-25 minutes

This Ayurvedic Apple Sauce with Ginger & Ghee is a delightful and nourishing breakfast option that incorporates warming spices and the digestive benefits of ghee. Adjust the sweetness and consistency according to your taste preferences and dosha considerations for a wholesome start to your day.

5. Ayurvedic Greens & Fresh Herb Frittata

Ingredients:

✓ 6 large eggs

✓ 1 cup spinach, chopped

✓ 1/2 cup kale, chopped

✓ 1/4 cup fresh cilantro, chopped

✓ 1/4 cup fresh parsley, chopped

✓ 1/4 cup fresh dill, chopped

✓ 1/2 cup onion, finely diced

✓ 1/2 cup zucchini, grated

✓ 1/2 cup bell peppers (any color), diced

✓ 1 tablespoon ghee or olive oil

✓ 1/2 teaspoon cumin seeds

✓ 1/2 teaspoon turmeric powder

✓ Salt and pepper to taste

Preparation:

1. Preheat your oven to 375°F (190°C).

2. In an oven-safe skillet, heat ghee or olive oil over medium heat.

3. Allow the cumin seeds to crackle for a few seconds before adding them.

4. Add diced onions, grated zucchini, and diced bell peppers.

5. Sauté until vegetables are softened.

6. Stir in chopped spinach, kale, cilantro, parsley, and dill.

7. Cook for another 2-3 minutes, or until the greens are wilted.

8. Whisk the eggs in a mixing basin until completely combined.

9. Add turmeric powder, salt, and pepper to the beaten eggs. Mix thoroughly.

10. Pour the beaten egg mixture into the skillet over the sautéed vegetables and greens.

11. Stir carefully to ensure that the ingredients are spread evenly.

12. Transfer the skillet to the preheated oven.

13. Bake for 15-20 minutes, or until the frittata is set and golden brown on top.

14. Once cooked, remove the frittata from the oven.

15. Garnish with additional fresh herbs if desired.

Total Nutritional Value (Approximate) for the entire Frittata: Total Calories: 272-276, Total Fat: 20.4-21.4g, Saturated Fat: 8g (from eggs and cooking oil), Total Protein: 11.9g,, Total Carbohydrates: 16.3g, Dietary Fiber: 4.4g, Total Sugars: 7.2g.

Preparation Time: 15 minutes

Cooking Time: 20-25 minutes

This Ayurvedic Greens & Fresh Herb Frittata is a nutrient-packed breakfast that combines the goodness of eggs, leafy greens, and aromatic herbs. Enjoy the vibrant flavors and nourishing benefits to kickstart your day. Adjust ingredient quantities based on personal preferences and dosha considerations for a wholesome and balanced meal.

6. Sweet Potato, Kale, and Black Bean Bowl

Ingredients:

✓ 1 large sweet potato, peeled and diced

✓ 1 cup kale, chopped

✓ 1 cup of black beans, cooked (canned or pre-cooked)

✓ 1 tablespoon ghee or olive oil

✓ 1/2 teaspoon cumin seeds

✓ 1/2 teaspoon coriander powder

✓ 1/2 teaspoon turmeric powder

✓ 1/2 teaspoon smoked paprika

✓ Salt and pepper to taste

✓ Fresh cilantro for garnish (optional)

✓ 1 tablespoon pumpkin seeds for garnish (optional)

✓ 1 tablespoon plain yogurt for serving (optional)

Preparation:

1. Preheat your oven to 400°F (200°C).

2. Toss the diced sweet potatoes with olive oil or ghee, cumin seeds, coriander powder, turmeric powder, smoked paprika, salt, and pepper.

3. Spread the seasoned sweet potatoes in a single layer on a baking pan.

4. Roast in the preheated oven for 20-25 minutes or until tender and golden brown, flipping halfway through.

5. In a skillet, heat ghee or olive oil over medium heat.

6. Add chopped kale and sauté until wilted and tender. Set aside.

7. In the same skillet, warm the cooked black beans.

8. You can add a pinch of cumin and salt for extra flavor.

9. In a bowl, layer the roasted sweet potatoes, sautéed kale, and warmed black beans.

10. Garnish with fresh cilantro and pumpkin seeds for added texture and nutritional value.

Total Nutritional Value (Approximate Per Serving): Calories: 588, Total Fat: 17g, Carbohydrates: 96.1g, Dietary Fiber: 24.9g, Protein: 22.4g.

Preparation Time: 15 minutes

Cooking Time: 25-30 minutes

This Ayurvedic Sweet Potato, Kale, and Black Bean Bowl provide a balance of flavors and nutrients, making it a wholesome and energizing breakfast option. Customize the bowl with your favorite toppings and enjoy the nourishing benefits of this Ayurvedic-inspired dish.

7. Ayurvedic Golden Milk Smoothie

Ingredients:

✓ 1 frozen banana, peeled and sliced

✓ 1/2 cup pineapple chunks

✓ 1/2 teaspoon ground turmeric

✓ 1/4 teaspoon ground ginger

✓ 1/4 teaspoon ground cinnamon

✓ 1/4 teaspoon black pepper

✓ 1 cup of almond milk (or your preferred milk)

✓ 1 tablespoon chia seeds

✓ 1 tablespoon almond butter

✓ 1 tablespoon of honey or maple syrup (optional, for additional flavor)

✓ Ice cubes (optional)

Preparation:

1. Peel and slice the banana. Measure out pineapple chunks, almond milk, chia seeds, and almond butter.

2. In a blender, combine the frozen banana slices, pineapple chunks, ground turmeric, ground ginger, ground cinnamon, black pepper, almond milk, chia seeds, and almond butter.

3. Combine the ingredients in a blender and process until smooth and creamy.

4. For a colder texture, add ice cubes and mix again..

5. Taste the smoothie and add honey or maple syrup if additional sweetness is desired. Blend again to incorporate.

6. Fill a glass halfway with the Golden Milk Smoothie.

Total Nutritional Value (Approximate per Serving): Calories: 405-407, Total Fat: 17.1-17.5g, Carbohydrates: 64.5-66.5g, Dietary Fiber: 16.9g, Sugars: 35.8-37.8g, Protein: 9.1-9.5g.

Preparation Time: 5 minutes

Blending Time: 3 minutes

This Ayurvedic Golden Milk Smoothie is a delightful and nutritious way to incorporate the healing properties of turmeric and other spices into your breakfast routine. Enjoy the smoothie for a refreshing start to your day, promoting balance and well-being. Adjust ingredients based on your dosha or personal preferences.

8. Date-Plum Cream

Ingredients:

✓ 1 cup ripe date-plums (jujubes), pitted

✓ 1/2 cup coconut cream

✓ 1 tablespoon chia seeds

✓ 1 teaspoon rose water

✓ 1/2 teaspoon ground cardamom

✓ 1 tablespoon chopped pistachios (for garnish)

✓ Fresh mint leaves (for garnish)

Preparation:

1. Wash and pit the date-plums.

2. You may use them whole if they are little.

3. If they are large enough, cut them into halves.

4. In a small bowl, soak chia seeds in 2 tablespoons of water for about 15 minutes until they form a gel-like consistency.

5. In a blender, combine ripe date-plums, coconut cream, soaked chia seeds, rose water, and ground cardamom.

6. Mix the ingredients until they are creamy and smooth.

7. If the cream is too thick, you can add a little water or more coconut cream to reach your desired consistency.

8. Transfer the date-plum cream to a bowl and refrigerate for at least 30 minutes to allow it to chill and enhance the flavors..

9. Before serving, garnish the date-plum cream with chopped pistachios and fresh mint leaves.

Total Nutritional Value (Approximate per Serving): Calories: 568, Total Fat: 39.9g, Carbohydrates: 49g, Dietary Fiber: 16.7g, Sugars: 29g, Protein: 7.7g

Preparation Time: 15 minutes

Chilling Time: 30 minutes

This Ayurvedic Date-Plum Cream is a delightful and naturally sweetened breakfast option that combines the unique flavors of date-plums with the richness of coconut cream. Enjoy this creamy and nourishing dish as a part of your Ayurvedic breakfast routine. Adjust ingredients based on your dosha or personal preference

9. Cauliflower and Fennel with Pumpkin Seeds

Ingredients:

✓ 1 medium-sized cauliflower, cut into florets

✓ 1 large fennel bulb, thinly sliced

✓ 2 tablespoons ghee or coconut oil

✓ 1 teaspoon cumin seeds

✓ 1 teaspoon coriander powder

✓ 1/2 teaspoon turmeric powder

✓ 1/2 teaspoon fennel seeds

✓ 1/4 cup pumpkin seeds

✓ Salt to taste

✓ Fresh cilantro for garnish (optional)

Preparation:

1. Cut the cauliflower into small florets.

2. Thinly slice the fennel bulb.

3. In a dry pan, toast the pumpkin seeds over medium heat until they are golden brown. Set aside.

4. In a large skillet, heat ghee or coconut oil over medium heat.

5. To the boiling oil, add cumin and fennel seeds.

6. Allow for a few seconds of sizzling.

7. Add cauliflower florets and sliced fennel to the skillet.

8. Sauté for 5-7 minutes until the vegetables are slightly tender but still crisp.

9. Sprinkle coriander powder, turmeric powder, and salt over the vegetables. Stir well to coat.

10. Cover the skillet and let the vegetables cook for an additional 5-7 minutes or until they reach your desired tenderness.

11. Stir in the toasted pumpkin seeds and cook for an additional 2 minutes.

12. Garnish with fresh cilantro just before serving if preferred.

13. **Total Nutritional Value (Approximate per Serving):** Calories: 639, Total Fat: 44g, Carbohydrates: 54g, Dietary Fiber: 20.5g, Sugars: 21g, Protein: 24g.

Preparation Time: 15 minutes

Cooking Time: 20 minutes

This Ayurvedic Cauliflower and Fennel with Pumpkin Seeds recipe is a delightful combination of flavors and textures, providing a nutritious and balanced breakfast. Enjoy the dish as a part of your Ayurvedic breakfast routine, incorporating the goodness of cauliflower, fennel, and pumpkin seeds. Adjust ingredients based on your dosha or personal preferences.

Balancing Doshas in the Morning Vata Dosha Breakfast

10. Baked Sweet Potato

Ingredients:

✓ 2 medium-sized sweet potatoes

✓ 1 tablespoon ghee or coconut oil

✓ 1 teaspoon ground cinnamon

✓ 1/2 teaspoon ground cardamom

✓ 1/2 teaspoon turmeric powder

✓ 1/4 teaspoon nutmeg

✓ A pinch of sea salt

✓ 1 tablespoon chopped nuts (such as almonds or walnuts, optional)

✓ 1 tablespoon dried cranberries or raisins (optional)

✓ Fresh mint leaves for garnish (optional)

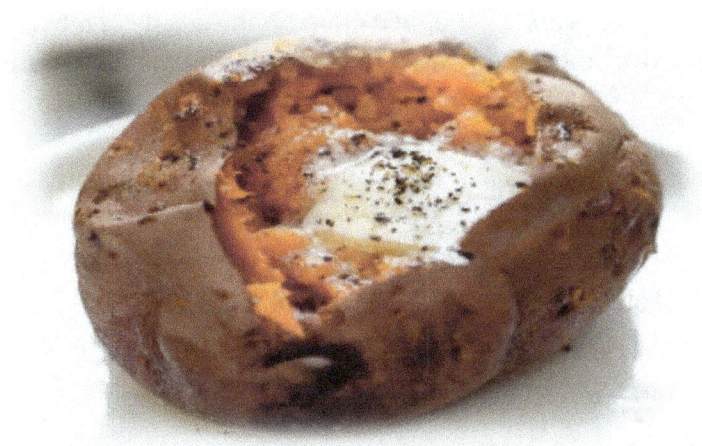

Preparation:

1. Preheat your oven to 400°F (200°C).

2. Wash and scrub the sweet potatoes thoroughly.

3. Cut each sweet potato in half lengthwise.

4. In a small bowl, mix together ground cinnamon, ground cardamom, turmeric powder, nutmeg, and a pinch of sea salt.

5. Brush each sweet potato half with ghee or coconut oil, ensuring they are well-coated.

6. Sprinkle the spice mixture evenly over the sweet potatoes, making sure to cover both the flesh and skin.

7. Line a baking sheet with parchment paper and place the seasoned sweet potatoes on it.

8. Bake in the preheated oven for 40-45 minutes or until the sweet potatoes are tender and can be easily pierced with a fork.

9. Optional: Sprinkle chopped nuts and dried cranberries or raisins over the baked sweet potatoes during the last 10 minutes of baking for added texture and sweetness.

10. Remove the roasted sweet potatoes from the oven.

11. Garnish with fresh mint leaves if desired.

Total Nutritional Value (Approximate per Serving): Calories: 303-323, Total Fat: 18.2-19.2g, Carbohydrates: 34-38g, Dietary Fiber: 3.8g, Protein: 3.3-4.3g.

Preparation Time: 10 minutes

Cooking Time: 40-45 minutes

This Ayurvedic Baked Sweet Potato recipe provides a warm and nourishing breakfast option rich in flavor and beneficial spices. Enjoy the natural sweetness of sweet potatoes and the added warmth of Ayurvedic spices to kickstart your day with a wholesome and satisfying meal.

Pitta Dosha Breakfast

11. Ayurvedic Egg Breakfast

Ingredients:

✓ 2 large eggs

✓ 1 tablespoon ghee or coconut oil

✓ 1/2 teaspoon cumin seeds

✓ 1/2 teaspoon turmeric powder

✓ 1/2 teaspoon ground coriander

✓ 1/4 teaspoon black pepper

✓ 1/4 teaspoon rock salt or sea salt

✓ 1/4 cup bell peppers, diced

✓ 1/4 cup spinach, chopped

✓ 1 tablespoon fresh cilantro, chopped (for garnish)

✓ 1 tablespoon plain yogurt (optional, for serving)

Preparation:

1. Dice bell peppers and chop spinach.

2. In a pan, heat ghee or coconut oil over medium heat.

3. Add cumin seeds to the heated oil and let them sizzle for a few seconds.

4. Add diced bell peppers to the pan and sauté until slightly softened.

5. Sprinkle turmeric powder, ground coriander, black pepper, and salt over the vegetables. Stir to combine.

6. Cook, stirring occasionally, until the spinach has wilted in the pan.

7. Create space in the pan and crack two eggs into the center.

8. Allow the eggs to cook undisturbed for a minute, then gently stir to scramble them with the vegetables.

9. Remove the pan from the heat after the eggs are done to your preference.

10. Garnish with fresh cilantro.

11. Optional: Serve the Ayurvedic egg breakfast with a dollop of plain yogurt on the side.

Total Nutritional Value (Approximate per Serving): Calories: 285, Total Fat: 25.7g, Protein: 13.7g, Carbohydrates: 5.9g, Dietary Fiber: 1.4g.

Preparation Time: 10 minutes

Cooking Time: 10 minutes

This Ayurvedic Egg Breakfast is a flavorful and protein-packed way to start your day, incorporating Ayurvedic spices for added warmth and digestive benefits. Adjust the spice levels and ingredients based on your dosha or personal preferences for a satisfying and balanced breakfast.

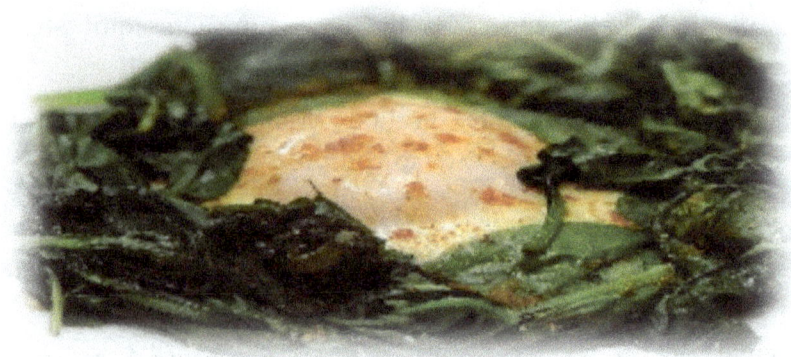

Kapha Dosha Breakfast

12. Breakfast Porridge with Rice Flake

Ingredients:

✓ 1/2 cup rice flakes (poha)

✓ 1 cup water

✓ 1/2 cup milk (dairy or plant-based)

✓ 1 tablespoon ghee

✓ 1/4 teaspoon ground cardamom

✓ 1/4 teaspoon ground cinnamon

✓ 1 tablespoon jaggery or honey (adjust to taste)

✓ 1 tablespoon of diced nuts (almonds, cashews, or pistachios)

✓ 1 tablespoon raisins

✓ Fresh fruits for topping (optional)

Preparation:

1. Rinse rice flakes under cold water to remove any impurities. Drain well.

2. Place rice flakes in a bowl and soak them in water for 5 minutes. Drain excess water.

3. In a saucepan over average heat, melt the ghee.

4. Add soaked rice flakes to the pan and sauté for 2-3 minutes until they become slightly crispy.

5. Pour 1 cup of water into the pan, followed by 1/2 cup of milk.

6. Bring to a slow boil, stirring constantly.

7. Add ground cardamom and ground cinnamon to the boiling mixture.

8. Reduce the heat and let it simmer until the rice flakes are fully cooked and the porridge reaches your desired consistency.

9. Stir in jaggery or honey to sweeten the porridge.

10. Adjust the sweetness to your preference.

11. Add chopped nuts (almonds, cashews, or pistachios) and raisins to the porridge.

12. Allow them to cook for an additional 2-3 minutes until the nuts are toasted and the raisins are plump.

13. Remove the porridge from heat.

14. Optionally, top with fresh fruits like sliced bananas or berries.

Total Nutritional Value (Approximate per Serving): Calories: 409-424, Total Fat: 21.5-22.5g, Carbohydrates: 49.5-54.5g, Protein: 11.8-12.8g.

Preparation Time: 10 minutes

Cooking Time: 15-20 minutes

This Ayurvedic Rice Flake Porridge is a wholesome and nourishing breakfast, combining the lightness of rice flakes with the richness of nuts and the sweetness of jaggery or honey. Adjust the ingredients based on your dosha or personal preferences for a delightful start to your day.

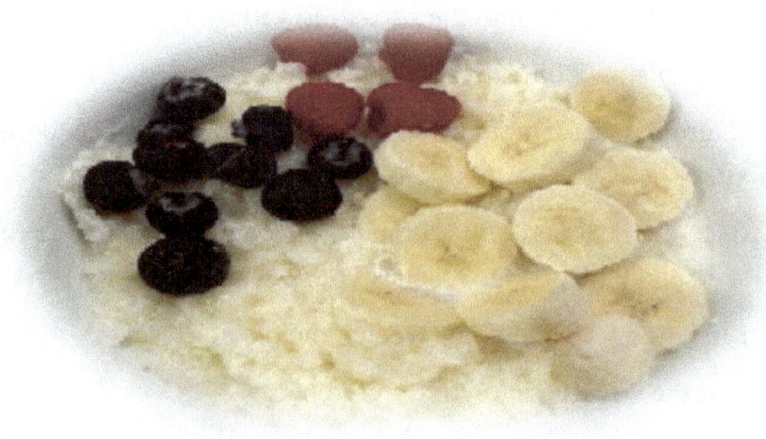

CHAPTER 4

WHOLESOME NOURISHING AYURVEDIC LUNCH RECIPES

1. Creamy Green Protein Soup for Pitta Dosha

Ingredients:

- ✓ 1 cup green split mung beans, soaked
- ✓ 1 cup zucchini, chopped
- ✓ 1 cup spinach leaves, chopped
- ✓ 1/2 cup fresh cilantro, chopped
- ✓ 1/2 cup fresh mint leaves
- ✓ 1/4 cup coconut cream
- ✓ 1 teaspoon ghee or coconut oil
- ✓ 1 teaspoon cumin seeds
- ✓ 1/2 teaspoon coriander powder
- ✓ 1/2 teaspoon fennel seeds
- ✓ 1/4 teaspoon turmeric powder
- ✓ 1/4 teaspoon ground black pepper
- ✓ 4 cups water or vegetable broth
- ✓ Salt to taste
- ✓ Squeeze of fresh lime juice (optional, for serving)

Preparation:

1. Rinse the green split mung beans and soak them in water for at least 4 hours or overnight. Drain before using.

2. Chop zucchini, spinach leaves, fresh cilantro, and mint leaves.

3. In a large pot, combine soaked mung beans and 4 cups of water or vegetable broth.

4. Bring to a boil, then reduce heat and simmer until the mung beans are soft and cooked through (approximately 20-25 minutes).

5. In a separate pan, heat ghee or coconut oil over medium heat.

6. Add cumin seeds, fennel seeds, coriander powder, turmeric powder, and ground black pepper.

7. Sauté for a minute until the spices release their aroma.

8. Add chopped zucchini to the sautéed spices and cook until slightly tender.

9. Once the mung beans are cooked, add the sautéed spices and zucchini to the pot.

10. Use an immersion blender to blend the soup until smooth and creamy.

11. Stir in chopped spinach, fresh cilantro, and mint leaves.

12. Cook for an additional 5 minutes until the greens are wilted.

13. Add coconut cream to the soup and stir well.

14. Season with salt to taste.

Total Nutritional Value (Approximate per Serving): Calories: 359, Total Fat: 13.1g, Carbohydrates: 46.6g, Dietary Fiber: 18.2g, Sugars: 7.6g, Protein: 17.4g.

Preparation Time: 15 minutes

Cooking Time: 30 minutes

This Ayurvedic Creamy Green Protein Soup is specially crafted for Pitta dosha, incorporating cooling and soothing ingredients. Enjoy the nourishing and balancing effects of this soup, perfect for a comforting dinner. Adjust ingredients based on your dosha or personal preferences.

2. Turmeric Lemon Rice for All Doshas

Ingredients:

✓ 1 cup basmati rice

✓ 2 cups water

✓ 1 tablespoon ghee or sesame oil

✓ 1 teaspoon mustard seeds

✓ 1 teaspoon cumin seeds

✓ 1/2 teaspoon turmeric powder

✓ 1/4 teaspoon asafoetida (hing)

✓ 1/2 cup cashews, chopped

✓ 1/4 cup fresh curry leaves

✓ 1 tablespoon ginger, finely grated

✓ 1 coarsely chopped green chile (adjust to taste)

✓ 1/4 cup lemon juice

✓ Salt to taste

✓ Fresh cilantro for garnish (optional)

Preparation:

1. Rinse basmati rice under cold water until the water flows is clean.

2. In a rice cooker or on the stovetop, cook the rice with 2 cups of water until fully done.

3. In a large pan, heat ghee or sesame oil over medium heat.

4. Mix in the mustard seeds, cumin seeds, turmeric powder, and asafoetida.

5. Give them a minute to sizzle.

6. Add chopped cashews to the pan and toast until they turn golden brown.

7. Add fresh curry leaves, grated ginger, and chopped green chili to the pan. Sauté for 2-3 minutes until fragrant.

8. Add the cooked basmati rice to the pan and gently mix, ensuring the rice is coated with the aromatic spices.

9. Drizzle lemon juice over the rice and mix well.

10. You can adjust the amount of lemon juice to your preference.

11. Season with salt to taste and continue to stir the rice, ensuring even distribution of flavors.

12. Garnish with fresh cilantro if desired for extra flavor.

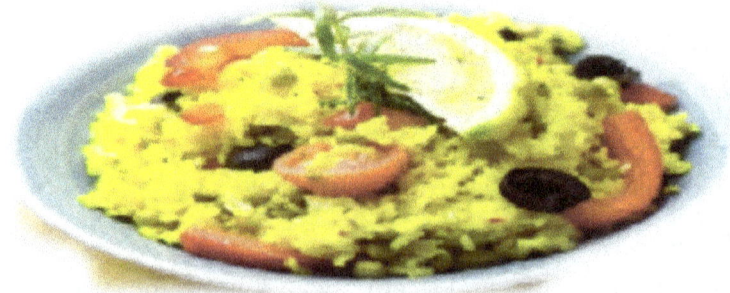

Total Nutritional Value (Approximate per Serving): Calories: 592, Total Fat: 32.2g, Carbohydrates: 65.5g, Dietary Fiber: 3.5g, Sugars: 4.5g, Protein: 15.3g

Preparation Time: 10 minutes

Cooking Time: 20 minutes

This Ayurvedic Turmeric Lemon Rice is a versatile and dosha-balancing dish suitable for all body types. Enjoy the vibrant flavors of turmeric and lemon, combined with the richness of cashews, for a wholesome and nourishing dinner. Adjust ingredients based on your dosha or personal preferences.

3. Ayurvedic Kitchari with Cilantro and Coconut

Ingredients:

✓ 1 cup basmati rice

✓ 1/2 cup yellow split mung beans

✓ 6 cups water

✓ 1 tablespoon ghee or sesame oil

✓ 1 teaspoon cumin seeds

✓ 1 teaspoon coriander powder

✓ 1/2 teaspoon turmeric powder

✓ 1/2 teaspoon mustard seeds

✓ 1/4 teaspoon asafoetida (hing)

✓ 1 cup mixed vegetables (carrots, peas, zucchini), chopped

✓ 1 tablespoon fresh ginger, grated

✓ 1 tablespoon fresh cilantro, chopped

✓ 1/2 cup coconut milk

✓ Salt to taste

✓ Fresh lime wedges for serving

Preparation:

1. Rinse basmati rice and yellow split mung beans under cold water until the water runs clear.

2. In a large pot, combine rice, yellow split mung beans, and 6 cups of water.

3. Bring to a boil, then reduce heat and simmer until both rice and mung beans are fully cooked (approximately 20-25 minutes).

4. In a separate pan, heat ghee or sesame oil over medium heat.

5. Add cumin seeds, coriander powder, turmeric powder, mustard seeds, and asafoetida.

6. Give them a minute or so to sizzle.

7. Add the chopped mixed vegetables and grated ginger to the pan. Sauté for 5-7 minutes until the vegetables are tender.

8. Add the sautéed vegetables and spices to the pot with cooked rice and mung beans.

9. Stir in chopped cilantro and coconut milk. Mix well to combine.

10. Season the kitchari with salt to taste. Stir and let it simmer for an additional 5-10 minutes.

Total Nutritional Value (Approximate Per Serving): Calories: 522, Total Fat: 25g, Carbohydrates: 63.7g, Dietary Fiber: 9.7g, Sugars: 3g, Protein: 13.3g.

Preparation Time: 15 minutes

Cooking Time: 35-40 minutes

This Ayurvedic Kitchari with Cilantro and Coconut is a nourishing and balancing dish suitable for all doshas. Enjoy the comforting flavors and healing properties of this traditional Ayurvedic recipe. Adjust ingredients based on your dosha or personal preferences. Serve with fresh lime wedges for an extra burst of flavor.

4. Ayurvedic Healing Soup for Acid Reflux

Ingredients:

- ✓ 1 cup carrots, peeled and chopped
- ✓ 1 cup zucchini, chopped
- ✓ 1 cup celery, chopped
- ✓ 1 cup fennel bulb, sliced
- ✓ 1 cup kale, chopped
- ✓ 1 tablespoon ghee or coconut oil
- ✓ 1 teaspoon cumin seeds
- ✓ 1 teaspoon coriander powder
- ✓ 1/2 teaspoon turmeric powder
- ✓ 1/4 teaspoon asafoetida (hing)
- ✓ 4 cups vegetable broth
- ✓ 1 cup water
- ✓ Salt to taste
- ✓ Fresh parsley for garnish (optional)

Preparation:

1. Peel and chop carrots.
2. Chop zucchini, celery, fennel bulb, and kale.
3. Heat ghee or coconut oil in a large saucepan over average heat.
4. Add cumin seeds, coriander powder, turmeric powder, and asafoetida. Sauté for a minute until aromatic.
5. Add chopped carrots, zucchini, celery, fennel bulb, and kale to the pot.
6. Sauté for 5-7 minutes, or until the veggies begin to soften.

7. Pour vegetable broth and water into the pot. Bring to a boil.

8. Reduce the heat and let the soup simmer for 20-25 minutes or until the vegetables are fully cooked.

9. Season the soup with salt to taste.

10. Use an immersion blender to blend the soup until smooth and creamy. Alternatively, transfer small batches to a blender and blend until smooth. Be cautious with hot liquids.

11. If desired, garnish the soup with fresh parsley for added freshness.

Total Nutritional Value (Approximate Per Serving): Calories: 144, Total Fat: 1.4g, Carbohydrates: 31g, Dietary Fiber: 10.4g, Sugars: 13.8g, Protein: 6.4g.

Preparation Time: 15 minutes

Cooking Time: 30-35 minutes

This Ayurvedic Healing Soup for Acid Reflux is a gentle and soothing option for those seeking relief. The combination of digestive-friendly vegetables and Ayurvedic spices aims to provide comfort while promoting digestive health. Adjust ingredients based on your preferences and dietary needs.

5. Easy Indian-Inspired Kitchari Bowls for Vata Dosha

Ingredients:

For Kitchari:

✓ 1/2 cup yellow split mung beans

✓ 1/2 cup white basmati rice

- ✓ 4 cups water
- ✓ 1 tablespoon ghee
- ✓ 1 teaspoon cumin seeds
- ✓ 1 teaspoon coriander powder
- ✓ 1/2 teaspoon turmeric powder
- ✓ 1/4 teaspoon asafoetida (hing)
- ✓ 1/2 teaspoon ginger, grated
- ✓ 1/2 teaspoon fennel seeds
- ✓ 1/4 cup carrots, finely chopped
- ✓ 1/4 cup zucchini, finely chopped
- ✓ 1/4 cup butternut squash, finely chopped
- ✓ Salt to taste
- ✓ Fresh cilantro for garnish

For Topping:

- ✓ 1/4 cup cooked quinoa
- ✓ 1/4 cup steamed kale, chopped
- ✓ 1/4 cup roasted sweet potatoes, diced
- ✓ 1 tablespoon toasted pumpkin seeds
- ✓ 1 tablespoon coconut flakes
- ✓ 1 tablespoon lemon juice

Preparation:

1. Rinse yellow split mung beans and white basmati rice under cold water until the water runs clear.
2. In a pot, combine mung beans, rice, and 4 cups of water.

3. Bring to a boil, then reduce heat and simmer until both mung beans and rice are fully cooked (approximately 20-25 minutes).

4. Heat the ghee in a separate pan over average heat.

5. Combine cumin seeds, coriander powder, turmeric powder, asafoetida, grated ginger, and fennel seeds in a mixing bowl.

6. Cook for a minute, or until the spices begin to release their scent.

7. Add finely chopped carrots, zucchini, and butternut squash to the pan. Sauté for 5-7 minutes until the vegetables are tender.

8. Once the mung beans and rice are cooked, add the sautéed vegetables and aromatic spices to the pot. Mix well.

9. Season the kitchari with salt to taste. Stir and let it simmer for an additional 5-10 minutes.

10. Cook quinoa according to package instructions.

11. Steam kale until tender.

12. Roast sweet potatoes in the oven until golden brown.

13. Toast pumpkin seeds in a dry pan until they pop.

14. In serving bowls, layer the kitchari with cooked quinoa, steamed kale, roasted sweet potatoes, toasted pumpkin seeds, and coconut flakes.

15. Garnish the kitchari bowls with fresh cilantro and drizzle with lemon juice. Serve warm.

Total Nutritional Value (Approximate Per Serving): Calories: 505, Total Fat: 22.5g, Carbohydrates: 71.7g, Dietary Fiber: 14.3g, Sugars: 8.8g, Protein: 14.8g.

Preparation Time: 15 minutes

Cooking Time: 40-45 minutes

This Easy Indian-Inspired Kitchari Bowl for Vata Dosha is a nourishing and grounding meal. Enjoy the blend of flavors and textures, providing warmth and balance to the Vata dosha. Adjust ingredients based on your dosha or personal preferences. Serve with love and gratitude for a wholesome Ayurvedic experience.

6. Ayurvedic Kitchari: A Simple and Nourishing Harmony

Ingredients:

For Kitchari:

✓ 1 cup yellow split mung beans, rinsed

✓ 1 cup white basmati rice, rinsed

✓ 2 tablespoons ghee

✓ 1 teaspoon cumin seeds

✓ 1 teaspoon coriander powder

✓ 1/2 teaspoon turmeric powder

✓ 1/2 teaspoon mustard seeds

✓ 1/2 teaspoon fennel seeds

✓ 1/2 inch fresh ginger, grated

✓ 1/2 teaspoon asafoetida (hing)

✓ 6 cups water

✓ 1 teaspoon salt (adjust to taste)

✓ Fresh cilantro for garnish

For Topping (Optional):

✓ 1/2 cup steamed vegetables (carrots, peas, zucchini)

✓ 1/4 cup plain yogurt

✓ Lemon wedges

Preparation:

1. Rinse yellow split mung beans and white basmati rice under cold water until the water runs clear.

2. In a large pot, heat ghee over medium heat.

3. Add cumin seeds, coriander powder, turmeric powder, mustard seeds, fennel seeds, grated ginger, and asafoetida.

4. Cook for a minute, stirring constantly, until the spices unleash their scent.

5. Fill the saucepan halfway with washed mung beans and rice.

6. Stir in the spices to coat.

7. Pour in 6 cups of water and add salt. Stir well.

8. Bring the mixture to a boil, then reduce the heat to low, cover the pot, and simmer for 25-30 minutes or until the mung beans and rice are fully cooked and the consistency is porridge-like.

9. Garnish the kitchari with fresh cilantro.

10. Serve the kitchari as is or top it with steamed vegetables, a dollop of plain yogurt, and lemon wedges.

Total Nutritional Value (Approximate Per Serving): Calories: 548, Total Fat: 27.8g, Carbohydrates: 64g, Dietary Fiber: 8.6g, Sugars: 2.2g, Protein: 18.2g

Preparation Time: 10 minutes

Cooking Time: 30 minutes

This Ayurvedic Kitchari is a simple, dynamic synergy of mung beans, basmati rice, and digestive spices. It's a nourishing and easily digestible dish, promoting balance and well-being. Adjust ingredients based on your dosha or personal preferences. Serve warm and savor the comforting and healing essence of this traditional Ayurvedic recipe.

7. Spiced Poha for All Doshas

Ingredients:

✓ 1 cup flattened rice (poha)

✓ 1/2 cup mixed vegetables (peas, carrots, and bell peppers), finely chopped

✓ 1 tablespoon ghee or coconut oil

✓ 1 teaspoon mustard seeds

✓ 1 teaspoon cumin seeds

✓ 1/4 teaspoon asafoetida (hing)

✓ 8-10 curry leaves

✓ 1 coarsely chopped green chile (adjust to taste)

✓ 1/2 cup peanuts, roasted

✓ 1/4 cup fresh coriander, chopped

✓ 1/2 teaspoon turmeric powder

✓ 1/2 teaspoon red chili powder (modify according to taste)

✓ Salt to taste

✓ Fresh lemon wedges for serving

Preparation:

1. Rinse the flattened rice under cold water. Drain and set aside.

2. In a pan, dry roast the peanuts until they are lightly browned. Set aside.

3. Cut the mixed veggies into tiny pieces using a fine knife.

4. In a large pan, heat ghee or coconut oil over medium heat.

5. Add mustard seeds, cumin seeds, asafoetida, and curry leaves. Allow them to splutter.

6. Add the finely chopped mixed veggies to the pan.

7. Cook for about 5-7 minutes, or until soft.

8. Add turmeric powder and red chili powder to the vegetables.

9. Mix well to coat the vegetables with the spices.

10. Add the rinsed flattened rice to the pan. Mix gently to combine with the vegetables and spices.

11. Cook for an additional 5 minutes.

12. Stir in the roasted peanuts and fresh coriander. Mix well.

13. Season the spiced poha with salt to taste.

14. Cook for another 2-3 minutes, stirring occasionally.

15. Serve the spicy poha garnished with fresh coriander.

16. Serve straight immediately, with lemon slices on the side.

Total Nutritional Value (Approximate Per Serving): Calories: 682, Total Fat: 51.5g, Carbohydrates: 46.2g, Dietary Fiber: 8.9g, Sugars: 5.9g, Protein: 19.7g.

Preparation Time: 15 minutes

Cooking Time: 20 minutes

This Ayurvedic Spiced Poha is a delightful and dosha-balancing dish suitable for all body types. Enjoy the aromatic spices, crunchy peanuts, and fresh vegetables in this quick and nourishing recipe.

Adjust ingredients based on your dosha or personal preferences. Serve with a squeeze of fresh lemon for added brightness.

8. Mediterranean Summer Salad for All Doshas

Ingredients:

✓ 2 cups of mixed greens (spinach, arugula, or your favorite)

✓ 1 cup cherry tomatoes, halved

✓ 1 cucumber, diced

✓ 1/2 cup Kalamata olives, pitted and sliced

✓ 1/2 cup feta cheese, crumbled (optional)

✓ 1/4 cup red onion, thinly sliced

✓ 1/4 cup fresh parsley, chopped

For the Dressing:

✓ 3 tablespoons extra-virgin olive oil

✓ 1 tablespoon balsamic vinegar

✓ 1 teaspoon Dijon mustard

✓ 1 clove garlic, minced

✓ Salt and pepper to taste

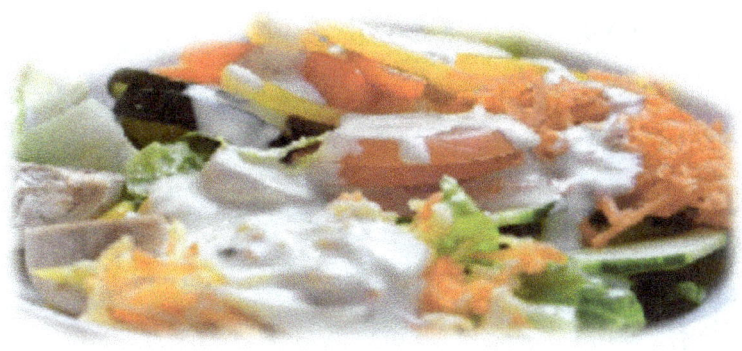

Preparation:

1. Wash and chop the mixed greens, cherry tomatoes, cucumber, Kalamata olives, red onion, and fresh parsley.

2. In a small bowl, whisk together extra-virgin olive oil, balsamic vinegar, Dijon mustard, minced garlic, salt, and pepper. Adjust the seasoning to taste.

3. In a large salad bowl, combine the mixed greens, cherry tomatoes, cucumber, Kalamata olives, red onion, and fresh parsley.

4. If using, crumble the feta cheese over the salad.

5. Pour the prepared dressing over the salad.

6. Gently toss the salad to ensure all ingredients are well coated with the dressing.

Total Nutritional Value (Approximate Per Serving): Calories: 869, Total Fat: 71.5g, Carbohydrates: 32.3g, Dietary Fiber: 8.4g, Sugars: 14.5g, Protein: 18.2g.

Preparation Time: 15 minutes

This Ayurvedic Mediterranean Summer Salad is a refreshing and balanced option for all doshas. Enjoy the vibrant flavors and nutritional benefits of this wholesome salad, perfect for a light and nourishing dinner. Adjust ingredients based on your dosha or personal preferences.

9. Roasted Tandoori Cauliflower Bowls for Kapha Dosha

Ingredients:

For Tandoori Cauliflower:

✓ 1 large cauliflower, cut into florets

✓ 2 tablespoons Greek yogurt

✓ 1 tablespoon chickpea flour (besan)

✓ 1 tablespoon tandoori spice mix

✓ 1 tablespoon ginger-garlic paste

✓ 1 tablespoon lemon juice

✓ 1 tablespoon olive oil

✓ 1 teaspoon cumin powder

✓ 1 teaspoon coriander powder

✓ 1/2 teaspoon turmeric powder

✓ Salt to taste

For Quinoa Base:

✓ 1 cup quinoa, rinsed

✓ 2 cups water

✓ 1/2 teaspoon cumin seeds

✓ 1/4 teaspoon turmeric powder

✓ 1 tablespoon ghee

For Toppings:

✓ 1 cup mixed greens (arugula, spinach, or kale)

✓ 1/2 cup cherry tomatoes, halved

✓ 1/4 cup red onion, thinly sliced

✓ 1/4 cup cucumber, diced

✓ 1/4 cup radishes, thinly sliced

✓ Fresh cilantro for garnish

✓ Lemon wedges for serving

Preparation:

1. Preheat the oven to 425°F (220°C).

2. In a bowl, mix Greek yogurt, chickpea flour, tandoori spice mix, ginger-garlic paste, lemon juice, olive oil, cumin powder, coriander powder, turmeric powder, and salt.

3. Coat cauliflower florets with the marinade.

4. Spread the cauliflower on a baking sheet lined with parchment paper.

5. Roast the cauliflower for 25 to 30 minutes in a preheated oven, or until it is soft and golden brown.

6. Heat ghee in a saucepan over a average heat.

7. Add cumin seeds and turmeric powder. Sauté for a minute until fragrant.

8. Add rinsed quinoa and sauté for another 2-3 minutes.

9. Pour in water, bring to a boil, then reduce heat to low, cover, and simmer for 15-20 minutes or until quinoa is cooked and water is absorbed.

10. In serving bowls, create a base with cooked quinoa.

11. Top with mixed greens, roasted tandoori cauliflower, cherry tomatoes, red onion, cucumber, and radishes.

12. Garnish the bowls with fresh cilantro and serve with lemon wedges on the side.

Total Nutritional Value (Approximate Per Serving): Calories: 317, Total Fat: 6.4g, Carbohydrates: 54.9g, Dietary Fiber: 10.7g, Sugars: 6.5g, Protein: 15.6g.

Preparation Time: 15 minutes

Cooking Time: 30-35 minutes

These Roasted Tandoori Cauliflower Bowls are designed to balance Kapha dosha, providing warmth, spice, and nutrient-dense ingredients. Enjoy the flavors and textures of this Ayurvedic-inspired dish, promoting harmony within the body. Adjust ingredients based on your dosha or personal preferences.

10. Easy One-Pot Lentil Kielbasa Soup for Pitta Dosha

Ingredients:

For Lentil Kielbasa Soup:

✓ 1 cup green or brown lentils, rinsed

✓ 1/2 pound (about 225g) kielbasa sausage, sliced

✓ 1 medium onion, diced

✓ 2 carrots, diced

✓ 2 celery stalks, diced

✓ 3 cloves garlic, minced

✓ 1 teaspoon cumin powder

✓ 1 teaspoon coriander powder

✓ 1/2 teaspoon turmeric powder

✓ 1/2 teaspoon fennel seeds

✓ 4 cups vegetable broth

✓ 2 cups water

✓ 1 bay leaf

✓ Salt and pepper to taste

✓ 2 tablespoons ghee or olive oil

✓ Fresh parsley for garnish

Preparation:

1. Rinse green or brown lentils under cold water until the water runs clear.
2. In a large pot, heat ghee or olive oil over medium heat.
3. Add diced onion, carrots, celery, and minced garlic. Sauté until vegetables are softened.
4. Add sliced kielbasa to the pot and sauté until lightly browned.
5. Add cumin powder, coriander powder, turmeric powder, and fennel seeds.
6. Stir the spices into the ingredients to coat them.
7. Add rinsed lentils, vegetable broth, water, and bay leaf to the pot.
8. Bring the soup to a boil, then reduce heat and simmer for about 25-30 minutes or until lentils are tender.
9. Add salt and pepper to the soup according to your to taste.
10. Garnish with fresh parsley for added freshness.

Total Nutritional Value (Approximate Per Serving): Calories: 942, Total Fat: 55.4g, Carbohydrates: 68.1g, Dietary Fiber: 26.4g, Sugars: 16.2g, Protein: 45.2g.

Preparation Time: 15 minutes

Cooking Time: 35-40 minutes

This Easy One-Pot Lentil Kielbasa Soup is designed to pacify Pitta dosha with its grounding and nourishing ingredients. Enjoy the comforting flavors of lentils and kielbasa in a balanced and soothing soup. Adjust ingredients based on your dosha or personal preferences. Serve warm and savor the simplicity and healthfulness of this Ayurvedic-inspired dish.

11. Ayurvedic Healing Kitchari for Recovery

Ingredients:

For Kitchari:

- ✓ 1 cup yellow split mung beans
- ✓ 1 cup white basmati rice
- ✓ 2 tablespoons ghee
- ✓ 1 teaspoon cumin seeds
- ✓ 1 teaspoon coriander powder
- ✓ 1/2 teaspoon turmeric powder
- ✓ 1/2 teaspoon mustard seeds
- ✓ 1/2 teaspoon fennel seeds
- ✓ 1/2 inch fresh ginger, grated
- ✓ 1/2 teaspoon asafoetida (hing)
- ✓ 6 cups water
- ✓ 1 teaspoon salt (adjust to taste)
- ✓ Fresh cilantro for garnish

For Topping (Optional):

- ✓ 1/2 cup steamed vegetables (carrots, peas, zucchini)
- ✓ 1/4 cup plain yogurt
- ✓ Lemon wedges

Preparation:

1. Rinse yellow split mung beans and white basmati rice under cold water until the water runs clear.

2. In a large pot, heat ghee over medium heat.

3. Add cumin seeds, coriander powder, turmeric powder, mustard seeds, fennel seeds, grated ginger, and asafoetida.

4. Cook for a minute, or until the spices begin to release their scent.

5. Pour in the washed mung beans and rice.

6. Toss to coat with the spices.

7. Pour in 6 cups of water and add salt. Stir well.

8. Bring the mixture to a boil, then reduce the heat to low, cover the pot, and simmer for 25-30 minutes or until the mung beans and rice are fully cooked and the consistency is porridge-like.

9. Garnish the kitchari with fresh cilantro.

10. Serve the kitchari as is or top it with steamed vegetables, a dollop of plain yogurt, and lemon wedges.

Total Nutritional Value (Approximate Per Serving): Calories: 548, Total Fat: 27.8g, Carbohydrates: 64g, Dietary Fiber: 8.6g, Sugars: 2.2g, Protein: 18.2g.

Preparation Time: 10 minutes

Cooking Time: 30 minutes

This Ayurvedic Healing Kitchari is a nourishing and easily digestible dish, perfect for healing and recovery. The combination of mung beans, rice, and Ayurvedic spices provides a balanced and comforting meal. Adjust ingredients based on your dosha or personal preferences. Serve warm and allow your body to benefit from the restorative properties of this traditional Ayurvedic dish.

12. Masala Rice (Vegetable Spiced Rice) for All Doshas

Ingredients:

✓ 1 cup basmati rice

✓ 2 cups of diced mixed veggies (carrots, peas, and bell peppers)

✓ 1 tablespoon ghee or sesame oil

✓ 1 teaspoon cumin seeds

✓ 1 teaspoon mustard seeds

✓ 1 teaspoon coriander powder

✓ 1/2 teaspoon turmeric powder

✓ 1/4 teaspoon asafoetida (hing)

✓ 1/2 teaspoon garam masala

✓ 1/4 teaspoon of red chili powder (adjust according to taste)

✓ Salt to taste

✓ Fresh cilantro for garnish

Preparation:

1. Basmati rice should be rinsed in cold water until the water is clean.

2. In a rice cooker or on the stovetop, cook the basmati rice with the appropriate amount of water until fully done.

3. Wash and chop the mixed vegetables into bite-sized pieces.

4. In a large pan, heat ghee or sesame oil over medium heat.

5. Add cumin seeds, mustard seeds, coriander powder, turmeric powder, asafoetida, garam masala, and red chili powder.

6. Cook for a minute, or until the spices begin to release their aroma.

7. Pour in the diced mixed veggies.

8. Sauté for 7-10 minutes until the vegetables are tender yet still vibrant.

9. Once the vegetables are cooked, add the cooked basmati rice to the pan. Mix well to ensure the rice is coated with the aromatic spices.

10. Season the masala rice with salt to taste.

11. Stir and let it cook for an additional 5 minutes, allowing the flavors to meld.

12. Garnish the masala rice with fresh cilantro for added freshness.

Total Nutritional Value (Approximate Per Serving): Calories: 391, Total Fat: 14.6g, Carbohydrates: 59.7g, Dietary Fiber: 6.3g, Sugars: 6g, Protein: 7.5g.

Preparation Time: 15 minutes

Cooking Time: 30 minutes

This Ayurvedic Masala Rice is a delightful and dosha-balancing dish suitable for all body types. Enjoy the aromatic blend of spices and the goodness of mixed vegetables in this wholesome and flavorful recipe. Adjust ingredients based on your dosha or personal preferences.

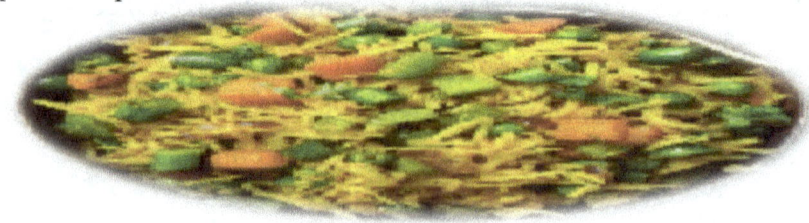

CHAPTER 5
AYURVEDIC DINNER RECIPES FOR DIGESTIVE EASE

1. Slow Cooker Quinoa Kichari

Ingredients:

For Quinoa Kichari:

- ✓ 1 cup split yellow mung dal, rinsed
- ✓ 1 cup quinoa, rinsed
- ✓ 1 cup mixed vegetables (carrots, peas, zucchini), chopped
- ✓ 1 large tomato, diced
- ✓ 1-inch piece of ginger, grated
- ✓ 2 teaspoons cumin powder
- ✓ 1 teaspoon coriander powder
- ✓ 1/2 teaspoon turmeric powder
- ✓ 1/2 teaspoon mustard seeds
- ✓ 1/2 teaspoon fennel seeds
- ✓ 4 cups vegetable broth
- ✓ 2 cups water
- ✓ 2 tablespoons ghee or coconut oil
- ✓ Salt to taste
- ✓ Fresh cilantro for garnish

For Tadka (Optional):

- ✓ 1 tablespoon ghee

✓ 1 teaspoon cumin seeds

✓ 1/2 teaspoon mustard seeds

✓ 1/4 teaspoon asafoetida (hing)

Preparation:

1. Rinse split yellow mung dal and quinoa under cold water until the water runs clear.

2. Chop mixed vegetables of your choice and dice the tomato.

3. In the slow cooker, combine rinsed mung dal, quinoa, mixed vegetables, diced tomato, grated ginger, cumin powder, coriander powder, turmeric powder, mustard seeds, fennel seeds, vegetable broth, water, and ghee or coconut oil. Add salt to taste.

4. Cover the slow cooker and set it to cook on low for 6-8 hours or until the dal and quinoa are cooked thoroughly and have a porridge-like consistency.

5. Heat ghee in a small saucepan over average heat.

6. Add cumin seeds, mustard seeds, and asafoetida. Allow the seeds to splutter.

7. Pour the tadka over the cooked kichari before serving for added flavor.

8. Garnish the kichari with fresh cilantro before serving.

Total Nutritional Value (Approximate Per Serving): Calories: 484, Total Fat: 4.7g, Carbohydrates: 89.4g, Dietary Fiber: 23.8g, Sugars: 9.4g, Protein: 23.3g.

Preparation Time: 15 minutes

Cooking Time: 6-8 hours in the slow cooker

This Slow Cooker Quinoa Kichari offers a convenient way to prepare a wholesome and balanced Ayurvedic meal. The slow cooking process allows the flavors to meld, resulting in a nourishing dish that supports digestion and overall well-being. Adjust ingredients based on your dosha or personal preferences. Serve warm and embrace the simplicity and healthfulness of this Ayurvedic-inspired recipe.

2. Hearty Vegetable Bean Soup

Ingredients:

✓ 1 cup mixed beans (kidney beans, chickpeas, lentils), soaked overnight

✓ 2 tablespoons ghee or olive oil

✓ 1 large onion, finely chopped

✓ 2 carrots, diced

✓ 2 celery stalks, diced

✓ 1 zucchini, diced

✓ 1 cup cabbage, shredded

✓ 3 tomatoes, diced

✓ 4 cups vegetable broth

✓ 4 cups water

✓ 1 teaspoon cumin powder

✓ 1 teaspoon coriander powder

✓ 1/2 teaspoon turmeric powder

✓ 1/2 teaspoon mustard seeds

✓ 1/2 teaspoon fennel seeds

✓ 2 bay leaves

✓ Salt and pepper to taste

✓ Fresh parsley for garnish

Preparation:

1. Soak mixed beans in water overnight.

2. In a large pot, heat ghee or olive oil over medium heat.

3. Add mustard seeds and fennel seeds. Allow them to splutter.

4. Add chopped onion and sauté until translucent.

5. Add diced carrots, celery, zucchini, and shredded cabbage.

6. Sauté for a few minutes until vegetables are slightly tender.

7. Add diced tomatoes to the pot.

8. Stir in cumin powder, coriander powder, turmeric powder, bay leaves, salt, and pepper. Mix well.

9. Drain and rinse the soaked beans.

10. Add the mixed beans to the pot.

11. Pour in vegetable broth and water. Stir to combine.

12. Bring the soup to a boil, then turn down to a low heat.

13. Cover the pot and simmer for about 45-60 minutes or until the beans are tender.

14. Taste the soup and adjust the seasoning if necessary.

15. Garnish the hearty vegetable bean soup with fresh parsley before serving.

Total Nutritional Value (Approximate Per Serving): Calories: 362, Total Fat: 2.6g, Carbohydrates: 70.4g, Dietary Fiber: 18g, Sugars: 12.6g, Protein: 16.5g.

Preparation Time: 15 minutes

Cooking Time: 45-60 minutes

Enjoy this nourishing and comforting Hearty Vegetable Bean Soup as a wholesome Ayurvedic lunch. Packed with a variety of beans and vegetables, it provides a balance of nutrients to support your well-being. Adjust ingredients based on your dosha or personal preferences. Serve warm and savor the goodness of this Ayurvedic-inspired recipe.

3. Basic Lassi, Sweet Lassi, and Salty Digestive Lassi

Ingredients:

For Basic Lassi:

✓ 1 cup plain yogurt

✓ 1/2 cup cold water

✓ 1 tablespoon honey or maple syrup (optional)

✓ Ice cubes (optional)

For Sweet Lassi:

✓ 1 cup plain yogurt

✓ 1/2 cup cold water

✓ 2 tablespoons honey or maple syrup

✓ 1/4 teaspoon cardamom powder

✓ Ice cubes (optional)

✓ Fresh mint leaves for garnish (optional)

For Salty Digestive Lassi:

✓ 1 cup plain yogurt

✓ 1/2 cup cold water

✓ 1/2 teaspoon cumin powder

✓ 1/4 teaspoon black salt

✓ Pinch of asafoetida (hing)

✓ Fresh coriander leaves for garnish (optional)

✓ Ice cubes (optional)

Preparation:

1. In a blender, combine the plain yogurt and cold water for each lassi variation.

2. Blend the yogurt and water until smooth.

3. If desired, sweeten with honey or maple syrup.

4. If desired, add ice cubes and blend again until frothy.

5. Pour into glasses and serve chilled.

6. Blend the yogurt, water, honey or maple syrup, and cardamom powder until smooth.

7. Add ice cubes if desired and blend again until frothy.and serve chilled.

8. Blend the yogurt, water, cumin powder, black salt, and a pinch of asafoetida until smooth.

9. Add ice cubes if desired and blend again until frothy.

10. Pour into glasses, garnish with fresh coriander leaves if desired, and serve chilled.

Total Nutritional Value (Approximate Per Serving): Vary based on chosen lassi variation

Basic Lassi: 5 minutes

Sweet Lassi: 7 minutes

Salty Digestive Lassi: 7 minutes

Serving Time: Immediate

Enjoy the refreshing goodness of these Ayurvedic Lassi variations. Whether you prefer the simplicity of Basic Lassi, the sweetness of Sweet Lassi, or the digestive benefits of Salty Digestive Lassi, these recipes provide a delightful way to incorporate Ayurvedic principles into your beverage choices. Adjust sweetness and spices according to your taste preferences. Serve chilled and embrace the soothing and balancing qualities of these traditional Ayurvedic drinks.

4. Fresh Homemade Yogurt or Ayurvedic Lassi

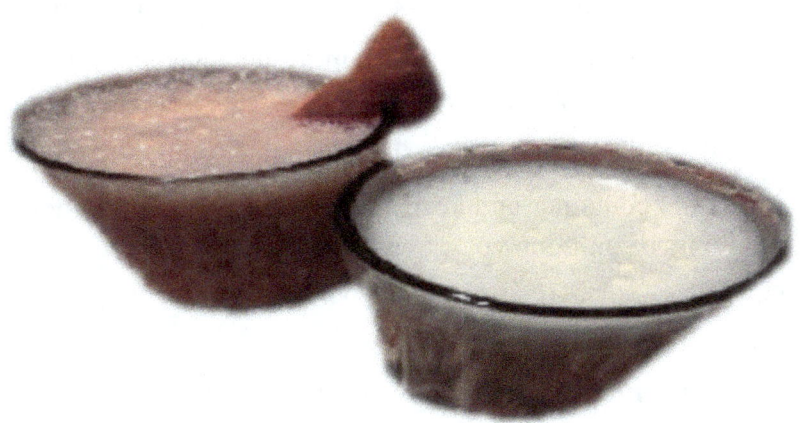

Ingredients:

✓ 1 quart (4 cups) whole milk

✓ 2 tablespoons of live and active cultures in plain yogurt

For Ayurvedic Lassi (Sweet or Salty):

✓ 1 cup fresh homemade yogurt

✓ 1/2 cup cold water

✓ 1 tablespoon honey or maple syrup (for Sweet Lassi)

✓ 1/2 teaspoon cumin powder (for Salty Lassi)

✓ 1/4 teaspoon black salt (for Salty Lassi)

✓ Ice cubes (optional)

✓ Fresh mint leaves for garnish (optional)

Preparation:

1. Heat the whole milk in a saucepan until it reaches just below boiling point (about 180°F or 82°C).

2. Allow the milk to cool to roughly 110°F (43°C).

3. In a small bowl, mix 2 tablespoons of plain yogurt with a few tablespoons of the cooled milk to create a smooth mixture.

4. Add the yogurt mixture back into the saucepan with the remaining milk and stir well.

5. Pour the milk mixture into a clean container with a lid.

6. Cover the container and keep it in a warm place to ferment for 6-8 hours or until the yogurt has set.

7. Once set, refrigerate the yogurt for at least 2 hours before using.

8. In a blender, combine 1 cup of fresh homemade yogurt and 1/2 cup of cold water.

9. For Sweet Lassi, add honey or maple syrup to the blender.

10. For Salty Lassi, add cumin powder and black salt to the blender.

11. Blend the mixture until smooth.

12. Add ice cubes if desired and blend again until frothy.

13. Pour into glasses, garnish with fresh mint leaves if desired, and serve chilled.

Total Nutritional Value (Approximate Per Serving - Ayurvedic Lassi): Varies based on chosen lassi variation

Fresh Homemade Yogurt: 10 minutes (plus fermentation time)

Ayurvedic Lassi: 5 minutes

Serving Time: Immediate

Adjust sweetness and spices according to your taste preferences for the Ayurvedic Lassi variations.

5. Clean Beets N Greens Kitchari

Ingredients:

✓ 1 cup basmati rice, rinsed

✓ 1/2 cup split yellow mung dal, rinsed

✓ 1 medium-sized beetroot, peeled and diced

✓ 2 cups mixed greens (spinach, kale, Swiss chard), chopped

✓ 1 small onion, finely chopped

✓ 2 cloves garlic, minced

✓ 1-inch piece of ginger, grated

✓ 1 teaspoon cumin seeds

✓ 1 teaspoon coriander powder

✓ 1/2 teaspoon turmeric powder

✓ 1/2 teaspoon mustard seeds

✓ 1/2 teaspoon fennel seeds

✓ 4 cups vegetable broth

✓ 2 cups water

✓ 2 tablespoons ghee or coconut oil

✓ Salt to taste

✓ Fresh cilantro for garnish

Preparation:

1. Rinse basmati rice and split yellow mung dal under cold water until the water runs clear.

2. Peel and dice the beetroot.

3. Chop mixed greens, onion, and garlic.

4. Heat ghee or coconut oil in a large saucepan over average heat.

5. Mix in the cumin, mustard, and fennel seeds.

6. Allow them to splutter.

7. Add chopped onion, garlic, and grated ginger.

8. Sauté until the onion is translucent.

9. Add diced beetroot and mixed greens to the pot.

10. Stir in coriander powder and turmeric powder. Mix well.

11. Add rinsed basmati rice and split yellow mung dal to the pot.

12. Stir until the ingredients are well combined.

13. Pour in vegetable broth and water. Add salt to taste. Stir well.

14. Bring the mixture to a boil, then reduce to a low temperature.

15. Cover the pot and simmer for 25-30 minutes or until the rice, dal, and vegetables are cooked and have a porridge-like consistency.

16. Garnish the Clean Beets N Greens Kitchari with fresh cilantro before serving.

Total Nutritional Value (Approximate Per Serving): Calories: 386, Total Fat: 1.3g, Carbohydrates: 81g, Dietary Fiber: 12.7g, Sugars: 11g, Protein: 15.5g.

Preparation Time: 15 minutes

Cooking Time: 25-30 minutes

Enjoy the nourishing and detoxifying benefits of this Clean Beets N Greens Kitchari. The combination of beets, greens, and spices in this Ayurvedic recipe provides a balanced and wholesome meal. Adjust spices and ingredients based on your dosha or personal preferences. Serve warm and embrace the vibrant flavors of this nutritious kitchari.

6. Quinoa Salad with Tangy Tahini Sauce

Ingredients:

For the Quinoa Salad:

✓ 1 cup quinoa, rinsed

✓ 2 cups water

✓ 1 cup cherry tomatoes, halved

✓ 1 cucumber, diced

✓ 1 bell pepper (any color), diced

✓ 1/4 cup red onion, finely chopped

✓ 1/4 cup fresh parsley, chopped

✓ 1/4 cup Kalamata olives, pitted and sliced

✓ 1/4 cup feta cheese, crumbled (optional)

✓ Salt and pepper to taste

For the Tangy Tahini Sauce:

✓ 1/4 cup tahini

- ✓ 2 tablespoons olive oil
- ✓ 2 tablespoons lemon juice
- ✓ 1 tablespoon apple cider vinegar
- ✓ 1 clove garlic, minced
- ✓ 1 teaspoon honey or maple syrup
- ✓ Salt and pepper to taste
- ✓ Water (to adjust consistency)

Preparation:

1. In a saucepan, combine quinoa and water.
2. Bring to a boil, then lower to a low heat, cover, and cook for 15-20 minutes, or until the quinoa is tender and the water has been absorbed.
3. Allow quinoa to cool before fluffing with a fork.
4. While quinoa is cooking, prepare the vegetables by chopping tomatoes, cucumber, bell pepper, red onion, parsley, and olives.
5. In a bowl, whisk together tahini, olive oil, lemon juice, apple cider vinegar, minced garlic, honey or maple syrup, salt, and pepper.
6. Add water gradually to achieve the desired sauce consistency.
7. Adjust salt and pepper to taste.
8. In a large bowl, combine cooked quinoa, chopped vegetables, and Kalamata olives.
9. Pour the tangy tahini sauce over the salad and toss until well coated.
10. If using, top with crumbled feta cheese.

11. Season with salt and pepper to taste.

12. Serve chilled or at room temperature.

Total Nutritional Value (Approximate Per Serving): Calories: 742, Total Fat: 55.6g, Carbohydrates: 46.4g, Dietary Fiber: 7.9g, Sugars: 2.5g, Protein: 19.1g.

Preparation Time: 20 minutes

Cooking Time: 15-20 minutes (for quinoa)

Enjoy the Quinoa Salad with Tangy Tahini Sauce as a wholesome and satisfying Ayurvedic lunch option, rich in protein, healthy fats, and fresh vegetables.

7. Saffron Rice

Ingredients:

✓ 1 cup basmati rice

✓ 2 cups water

✓ A pinch of saffron threads

✓ 2 tablespoons warm milk

✓ 1 tablespoon ghee or coconut oil

✓ 1/4 cup cashews, chopped

✓ 1/4 cup raisins

✓ 1 teaspoon cumin seeds

✓ 1 cinnamon stick

✓ 2-3 green cardamom pods

✓ Salt to taste

✓ Fresh cilantro for garnish (optional)

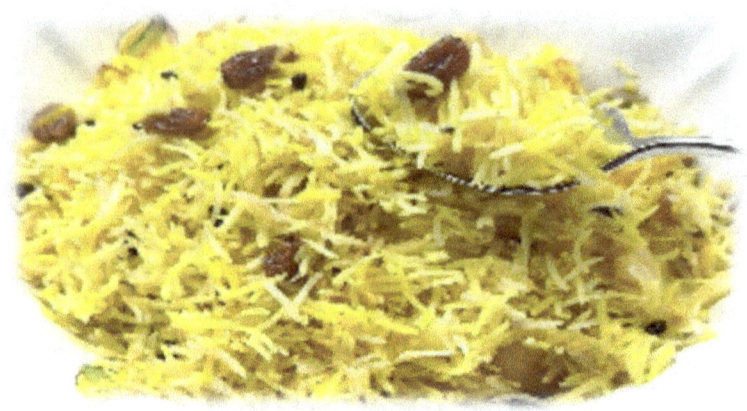

Preparation:

1. Basmati rice should be rinsed in cold water until the water is clean.

2. Set aside the saffron threads that have been soaked in heated milk.

3. 2 cups water, brought to a boil in a pot.

4. Add rinsed basmati rice to the boiling water.

5. Cook the rice on low heat until all the water is absorbed and the rice is tender. Fluff the rice with a fork.

6. Pour the saffron-soaked milk over the cooked rice and gently fold it in.

7. Allow the saffron to infuse its color and flavor into the rice.

8. In a separate pan, heat ghee or coconut oil over medium heat.

9. Add chopped cashews and raisins.

10. Sauté until the cashews are golden and the raisins are plump.

11. Add cumin seeds, cinnamon stick, and green cardamom pods to the pan with cashews and raisins.

12. Cook for a minute, or until the spices begin to release their scent.

13. Add the cooked rice to the pan with the sautéed cashews, raisins, and spices.

14. Gently mix everything together.

15. Season the saffron rice with salt to taste.

16. Garnish with fresh cilantro if desired.

Total Nutritional Value (Approximate Per Serving): Calories: 612, Total Fat: 28.6g, Carbohydrates: 83g, Dietary Fiber: 3.1g, Sugars: 18.2g, Protein: 10.2g.

Preparation Time: 15 minutes

Cooking Time: 20-25 minutes (for rice).

Serve the fragrant and vibrant Saffron Rice as a delightful side dish or as part of a balanced Ayurvedic meal. Enjoy the rich flavors and beautiful color of this dish that can complement a variety of main courses.

8. Upma (Savory Cream of Wheat)

Ingredients:

✓ 1 cup semolina (cream of wheat)

✓ 2 tablespoons ghee or coconut oil

✓ 1 teaspoon mustard seeds

✓ 1 teaspoon cumin seeds

✓ 1/2 cup chopped onions

✓ 1/4 cup chopped carrots

✓ 1/4 cup green peas

✓ 1/4 cup chopped bell peppers (any color)

✓ 1/4 cup chopped tomatoes

✓ 1 teaspoon grated ginger

✓ 2 green chilies, finely chopped

✓ 1/4 teaspoon turmeric powder

✓ 1/4 teaspoon asafoetida (hing)

✓ 2 1/2 cups water

✓ Salt to taste

✓ Fresh cilantro for garnish (optional)

✓ Lemon wedges for serving

Preparation:

1. Dry roast the semolina in a pan over medium heat until it turns golden brown.

2. Keep stirring to avoid burning. Set aside.

3. In a separate pan, heat ghee or coconut oil over medium heat.

4. Add mustard seeds and cumin seeds. Allow them to splutter.

5. Sauté the onions until they are transparent.

6. Toss in the carrots, green peas, bell peppers, tomatoes, grated ginger, and green chilies.

7. Cook for a few minutes, or until the veggies are soft.

8. Sprinkle turmeric powder and asafoetida over the vegetables. Mix well.

9. Add the roasted semolina to the pan. Mix it thoroughly with the sautéed vegetables.

10. In a steady stream, pour 2 1/2 cups of water into the pan while continuously stirring to avoid lumps.

11. Add salt to taste and continue stirring to ensure even cooking.

12. Reduce the heat to low, cover the pan, and let the Upma simmer.

13. Stir occasionally to prevent sticking.

14. Once the Upma has absorbed the water and reached a creamy consistency, remove it from heat.

15. Garnish with fresh cilantro if desired.

Total Nutritional Value (Approximate Per Serving): Varies based on serving size and specific ingredients

Preparation Time: 15 minutes

Cooking Time: 15-20 minutes

Serve the hot and flavorful Upma on plates, garnished with fresh cilantro and accompanied by lemon wedges. Enjoy this traditional Ayurvedic dish as a wholesome and satisfying lunch option.

9. Spiced Poha

Ingredients:

- ✓ 1 cup flattened rice (poha)
- ✓ 2 tablespoons ghee or coconut oil
- ✓ 1 teaspoon mustard seeds
- ✓ 1/2 teaspoon cumin seeds
- ✓ 1/2 cup chopped onions
- ✓ 1/4 cup green peas
- ✓ 1/4 cup chopped carrots
- ✓ 2 green chilies, finely chopped

- ✓ 1/2 teaspoon turmeric powder
- ✓ 1/2 teaspoon of red chili powder (modify according to taste)
- ✓ Salt to taste
- ✓ 1 tablespoon lemon juice
- ✓ Fresh cilantro for garnish
- ✓ 2 tablespoons roasted peanuts (optional)

Preparation:

1. In a strainer, rinse the flattened rice (poha) under cold water.
2. Allow it to soak for 5-7 minutes until it becomes soft but not mushy.
3. In a pan, heat ghee or coconut oil over medium heat.
4. Add mustard seeds and cumin seeds. Allow them to splutter.
5. Add chopped onions, green peas, and chopped carrots.
6. Sauté until the vegetables are tender.
7. Stir in chopped green chilies, turmeric powder, and red chili powder. Mix well.
8. Add the saturated and drained poha to the pan.
9. Gently toss to combine all the ingredients.
10. Cook for 3-5 minutes, stirring occasionally, until the poha is heated through and well-incorporated with the spices and vegetables.
11. Season the spiced poha with salt to taste.
12. Add lemon juice and mix well.
13. Garnish the spiced poha with fresh cilantro and, if desired, roasted peanuts for added crunch.

Total Nutritional Value (Approximate Per Serving): Varies based on serving size and specific ingredients.

Preparation Time: 10 minutes

Cooking Time: 10 minutes

Serve the warm and flavorful Spiced Poha on plates, garnished with fresh cilantro and, if desired, roasted peanuts. This quick and nutritious Ayurvedic lunch option is a perfect balance of carbohydrates, protein, and healthy fats. Enjoy the delicious blend of spices and textures in every bite.

10. Sage Gravy

Ingredients:

✓ 1/4 cup ghee

✓ 1/4 cup whole wheat flour

✓ 2 cups vegetable or chicken broth

✓ 1 tablespoon fresh sage leaves, finely chopped

✓ 1/2 teaspoon ground black pepper

✓ 1/2 teaspoon sea salt

✓ 1/2 teaspoon onion powder

✓ 1/2 teaspoon garlic powder

Preparation:

1. Finely chop fresh sage leaves.

2. Melt ghee in a pot over medium heat.

3. To make a roux, mix in the whole wheat flour continually.

4. Stir the roux and cook for 2 to 3 minutes, or until golden brown.

5. Slowly pour in the vegetable or chicken broth while whisking continuously to avoid lumps.

6. Add chopped sage, ground black pepper, sea salt, onion powder, and garlic powder. Stir well to combine.

7. Bring the mixture to a gentle simmer.

8. Reduce heat and let it cook for an additional 5-7 minutes, stirring occasionally until the gravy thickens.

9. If the gravy is too thick, you can add more broth to achieve the desired consistency.

Total Nutritional Value (ApproximateWhole Recipe): Calories: 588, Total Fat: 52g, Carbohydrates: 29g, Dietary Fiber: 4g, Sugars: 2g, Protein: 5g.

Preparation Time: 10 minutes

Cooking Time: 10-15 minutes

This Sage Gravy is a delightful addition to your festive celebrations. Serve it over roasted vegetables, mashed potatoes, or your favorite holiday dishes for a comforting and flavorful experience.

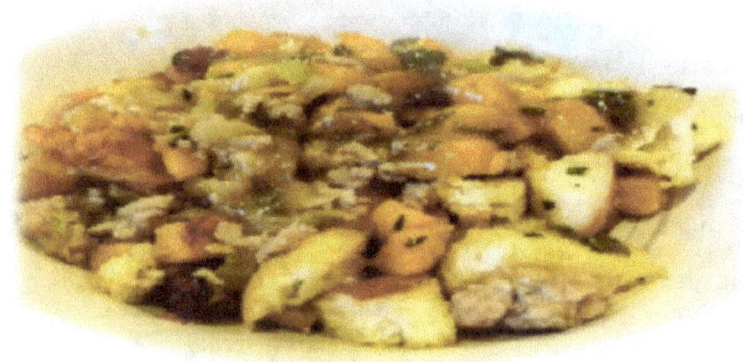

CHAPTER 6

AYURVEDIC SNACK IDEAS FOR BALANCED ENERGY

1. Coconut Milk, Chia Seed & Vanilla Bean Pudding

Ingredients:

- ✓ 1/4 cup chia seeds
- ✓ 1 can (14 oz) coconut milk
- ✓ 1-2 tablespoons of maple syrup or honey (modify to taste)
- ✓ 1 vanilla bean (or 1 teaspoon vanilla essence)
- ✓ Fresh fruits for topping (e.g., berries, sliced mango, or kiwi)

Preparation:

1. In a mixing bowl, combine the chia seeds and the coconut milk.
2. Mix carefully to ensure that the chia seeds are uniformly distributed.
3. Add maple syrup or honey to the chia seed mixture.
4. Adjust the sweetness to your liking.
5. If using a vanilla bean, split it lengthwise with a knife.
6. Scrape out the seeds with the back of a knife.
7. Add the extracted vanilla seeds (or vanilla extract if using) to the chia seed mixture.
8. Stir to infuse the pudding with a delightful vanilla flavor.

9. Cover the bowl and refrigerate the chia seed mixture for at least 4 hours or overnight.

10. The chia seeds will absorb the liquid and form a pudding-like consistency as a result.

11. Before serving, give the pudding a good stir to ensure an even texture.

Total Nutritional Value (Approximate Per Serving): Calories: 1020-1100 (varies based on sweetener quantity), Total Fat: 81g, Carbohydrates: 63g, Dietary Fiber: 10g, Sugars: 27g, Protein: 12g.

Preparation Time: 5 minutes

Refrigeration Time: 4 hours or overnight

Spoon the Coconut Milk, Chia Seed & Vanilla Bean Pudding into serving bowls or glasses. Top with fresh fruits such as berries, sliced mango, or kiwi for added freshness and flavor. Enjoy this wholesome Ayurvedic snack that combines the goodness of chia seeds, coconut milk, and natural sweetness.

2. Country-Home Sweet Potato & Spicy Pecan Crisp

Ingredients:

For the Filling:

✓ 3 medium-sized sweet potatoes, peeled and thinly sliced

✓ 1 cup chopped pecans

✓ 1/4 cup maple syrup

✓ 1/4 cup melted ghee or coconut oil

✓ 1 teaspoon ground cinnamon

✓ 1/2 teaspoon ground nutmeg

✓ 1/4 teaspoon ground ginger

✓ A pinch of salt

For the Topping:

✓ 1 cup old-fashioned rolled oats

✓ 1/2 cup almond flour

✓ 1/2 cup chopped pecans

✓ 1/4 cup maple syrup

✓ 1/4 cup melted ghee or coconut oil

✓ 1/2 teaspoon ground cinnamon

✓ A pinch of salt

Preparation:

1. Preheat your oven to 350°F (175°C).

2. In a large bowl, combine thinly sliced sweet potatoes, chopped pecans, maple syrup, melted ghee or coconut oil, ground cinnamon, ground nutmeg, ground ginger, and a pinch of salt.

3. Toss the mixture until the sweet potatoes are well coated.

4. Transfer the sweet potato mixture to a baking dish, spreading it evenly.

5. In a separate bowl, combine rolled oats, almond flour, chopped pecans, maple syrup, melted ghee or coconut oil, ground cinnamon, and a pinch of salt.

6. Mix until the ingredients are well combined.

7. Sprinkle the oat and pecan topping evenly over the sweet potato mixture in the baking dish.

8. Place the baking dish in the preheated oven and bake for approximately 40-45 minutes or until the sweet potatoes are tender, and the topping is golden brown.

Total Nutritional Value (Approximate Per Serving): Varies based on serving size and specific ingredients

Preparation Time: 15 minutes

Baking Time: 40-45 minutes

Allow the Country-Home Sweet Potato & Spicy Pecan Crisp to cool for a few minutes before serving. Enjoy this delightful and nourishing Ayurvedic snack with a perfect balance of sweet and savory flavors. Serve it as a comforting treat during cooler seasons or as a wholesome dessert option.

3. Ghee-Sautéed Bananas with Cinnamon and Ginger

Ingredients:

✓ 2 ripe bananas, sliced

✓ 2 tablespoons ghee

✓ 1 teaspoon ground cinnamon

✓ 1/2 teaspoon ground ginger

✓ Optional: Honey or maple syrup for drizzling

Preparation:

1. Peel and slice the ripe bananas into rounds.

2. In a skillet, heat 2 tablespoons of ghee over medium heat.

3. Add the banana slices to the skillet and sauté for 2-3 minutes on each side or until they become golden brown.

4. Sprinkle ground cinnamon and ground ginger over the sautéed bananas. Toss gently to coat the bananas evenly with the spices.

5. If desired, drizzle honey or maple syrup over the sautéed bananas for added sweetness. Toss gently to combine.

Total Nutritional Value (Approximate Per Serving): Calories: 523, Total Fat: 29g, Carbohydrates: 73.7g, Dietary Fiber: 7.1g, Sugars: 47.2g, Protein: 2.3g.

Preparation Time: 5 minutes

Cooking Time: 5-7 minutes

Serve the Ghee-Sautéed Bananas with Cinnamon and Ginger warm, either on their own or as a delightful topping for yogurt or oatmeal. This quick and easy Ayurvedic snack provides a balance of natural sweetness and warming spices, making it a nourishing and comforting treat.

4. Frothy Almond Date Shake

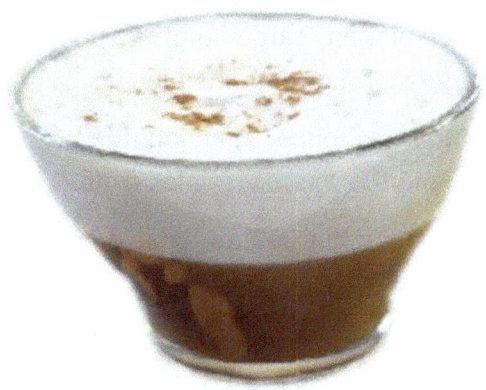

Ingredients:

✓ 1 cup almonds, soaked overnight

- ✓ 6-8 Medjool dates, pitted
- ✓ 2 cups milk (dairy or plant-based)
- ✓ 1/2 teaspoon ground cinnamon
- ✓ 1/4 teaspoon cardamom powder
- ✓ 1/2 teaspoon vanilla extract
- ✓ Ice cubes (optional)

Preparation:

1. Place almonds in a bowl and cover them with water. Allow them to soak overnight.

2. This softens the almonds and allows them to combine more easily.

3. Drain and rinse the almonds under cold water after soaking.

4. Blend soaked almonds, pitted dates, and milk in a blender.

5. Blend the contents until it is smooth and creamy.

6. Add ground cinnamon, cardamom powder, and vanilla extract to the almond-date mixture in the blender.

7. Blend the mixture once again until the spices are well incorporated, and the shake becomes frothy.

8. If you prefer a smoother texture, you can strain the shake using a fine mesh sieve or cheesecloth to remove almond pulp.

9. This step is optional, and you can skip it if you enjoy the fiber content.

10. If you like your shake chilled, you can add ice cubes to the blender and blend until they are crushed and the shake becomes cold.

Total Nutritional Value (Approximate Per Serving): Varies based on milk type and serving size

Soaking Time: Overnight

Preparation Time: 10 minutes

Pour the Frothy Almond Date Shake into glasses and enjoy the rich, nutty flavor with a hint of sweetness. This Ayurvedic snack provides a nutritious and energy-boosting option for a quick pick-me-up.

5. Apple Sauce with Ginger & Ghee

Ingredients:

✓ 4 medium-sized apples, peeled, cored, and diced

✓ 1 tablespoon ghee

✓ 1 teaspoon freshly grated ginger

✓ 1-2 tablespoons honey or maple syrup (optional, based on sweetness preference)

✓ 1/2 teaspoon ground cinnamon

✓ 1/4 cup water

Preparation:

1. The apples should be peeled, cored, and diced into tiny pieces.

2. In a saucepan, melt 1 tablespoon of ghee over medium heat.

3. Add the diced apples to the saucepan and sauté for 3-4 minutes until they start to soften.

4. Stir in the freshly grated ginger, ensuring it is well combined with the apples.

5. If desired, add honey or maple syrup to the apples for sweetness.

6. Adjust the quantity based on your preference.

7. Sprinkle ground cinnamon over the apples and stir to incorporate the spice.

8. Pour 1/4 cup of water into the saucepan to help the apples cook and create a sauce.

9. Reduce the heat to low, cover the saucepan, and let the apples simmer for 15-20 minutes or until they become tender.

10. Use a potato masher or an immersion blender to mash the cooked apples until you reach your desired consistency.

11. Blend it until smooth if you desire a smoother sauce.

Total Nutritional Value (Approximate)Per Serving): Calories: 532-596 (varies based on sweetener quantity), Total Fat: 16.1g, Carbohydrates: 108.2g, Dietary Fiber: 17.7g, Sugars: 85.2g, Protein: 1.2g.

Preparation Time: 10 minutes

Cooking Time: 20-25 minutes

Serve the Apple Sauce with Ginger & Ghee warm or chilled, as a delicious snack or a wholesome topping for pancakes, yogurt, or oatmeal. This Ayurvedic treat combines the natural sweetness of apples with the warmth of ginger and cinnamon, creating a comforting and nourishing snack option.

6. Fresh Ginger Tea with Raw Honey

Ingredients:

✓ 1 tablespoon fresh ginger, peeled and grated

✓ 2 cups water

✓ 1 tablespoon raw honey (adjust to taste)

✓ Optional: Lemon slices for garnish

Preparation:

1. Grate and peel one tablespoon of raw ginger.

2. In a small pot, boil two cups of water.

3. Over the grated ginger, pour the boiling water.

4. Reduce the heat to low, cover the saucepan, and let the ginger simmer in the water for 10-15 minutes to infuse its flavor.

5. After simmering, strain the ginger tea to remove the grated ginger pieces, leaving you with a clear tea.

6. While the tea is still warm, add 1 tablespoon of raw honey and stir until it dissolves.

7. Adjust the honey quantity based on your sweetness preference.

8. If desired, garnish the tea with lemon slices for a citrusy twist.

Total Nutritional Value (Approximate Per Serving): Calories: 68, Carbohydrates: 18g, Sugars: 17g, Protein: 0.1g.

Preparation Time: 5 minutes

Cooking Time: 15 minutes

Pour the Fresh Ginger Tea with Raw Honey into your favorite mug and enjoy this soothing and warming Ayurvedic snack. This tea not only provides comfort but also has potential health benefits, making it a delightful addition to your wellness routine.

7. Savory Turmeric-Spiced Popcorn

Ingredients:

✓ 1/2 cup popcorn kernels

✓ 3 tablespoons ghee

✓ 1 teaspoon ground turmeric

✓ 1/2 teaspoon ground cumin

✓ 1/2 teaspoon ground coriander

✓ 1/4 teaspoon cayenne pepper (adjust to taste)

✓ Salt to taste

Preparation:

1. Using your favorite technique (air popper, stovetop, or microwave), to pop the popcorn kernels.

2. In a small saucepan, melt 3 tablespoons of ghee over low heat.

3. In a small bowl, mix ground turmeric, ground cumin, ground coriander, cayenne pepper, and salt.

4. Pour the melted ghee over the popped popcorn and toss to coat evenly.

5. Sprinkle the spice mix over the popcorn and toss again to ensure even coating.

Total Nutritional Value (Approximate Per Serving): Calories: 617, Total Fat: 43.5g, Carbohydrates: 51.1g, Dietary Fiber: 14.2g, Sugars: 0.4g, Protein: 12.7g.

Preparation Time: 10 minutes (excluding popcorn popping time)

Enjoy the Savory Turmeric-Spiced Popcorn as a flavorful and wholesome Ayurvedic snack. This unique twist on popcorn adds the goodness of turmeric and spices, creating a delicious and satisfying treat.

8. Rice Cakes with Raw Kraut or Kimchi

Ingredients:

✓ 4 rice cakes

✓ 1 cup raw kraut or kimchi

✓ 2 tablespoons sesame seeds

✓ 1 tablespoon olive oil

✓ Fresh cilantro leaves for garnish (optional)

Preparation:

1. In a dry skillet over medium heat, toast 2 tablespoons of sesame seeds until golden brown. Set aside.

2. Toast 4 rice cakes to your liking.

3. Place the toasted rice cakes on a serving plate.

4. Spoon 1 cup of raw kraut or kimchi onto each rice cake.

5. Drizzle 1 tablespoon of olive oil over the kraut or kimchi-topped rice cakes.

6. Top with the toasted sesame seeds.

7. Garnish with fresh cilantro leaves for added flavor and a pop of color.

Nutritional Value (Per Serving): Calories: 564, Total Fat: 24g, Saturated Fat: 3g, Sodium: 880mg, Total Carbohydrates: 79g, Dietary Fiber: 6g, Sugars: 1g, Protein: 9g

Preparation Time: 10 minutes (excluding toasting time for rice cakes)

Enjoy these Rice Cakes with Raw Kraut or Kimchi as a delightful Ayurvedic snack. The combination of crispy rice cakes, tangy kraut or kimchi, and the nutty flavor of sesame seeds creates a flavorful and satisfying treat that's perfect for any time of day.

9. Baked Apple with Clove

Ingredients:

✓ 2 apples (preferably a sweet variety)

✓ 1 teaspoon ground cloves

✓ 1 tablespoon ghee

✓ 1 tablespoon honey or maple syrup (optional)

✓ chopped nuts for garnish, such as walnuts or almonds (optional)

Preparation:

1. Preheat the oven to 375°F (190°C).

2. Remove the seeds from the apples and make a hole in the center.

3. Sprinkle 1/2 teaspoon of ground cloves into the well of each apple.

4. Place 1/2 tablespoon of ghee on top of the cloves in each apple.

5. If desired, drizzle 1/2 tablespoon of honey or maple syrup over each apple for added sweetness.

6. Place the prepared apples in a baking dish and bake in the preheated oven for 25-30 minutes or until the apples are tender.

7. If desired, garnish with chopped nuts like almonds or walnuts for added texture.

Total Nutritional Value (Approximate Per Serving): Calories: 390, Total Fat: 16.3g, Saturated Fat: 9.3g, Trans Fat: 0g, Cholesterol: 37mg, Sodium: 4mg, Total Carbohydrates: 72.4g, Dietary Fiber: 11.7g, Sugars: 55.1g, Protein: 1.2g.

Preparation Time: 10 minutes

Baking Time: 25-30 minutes

Serve the Baked Apple with Clove warm as a delightful Ayurvedic snack. The combination of baked apple with aromatic cloves creates a comforting and flavorful treat, perfect for a nourishing snack or dessert.

10. Kitchari Snack

Ingredients:

✓ 1/2 cup yellow mung dal

✓ 1/2 cup basmati rice

✓ 1 tablespoon ghee

✓ 1 teaspoon cumin seeds

✓ 1/2 teaspoon mustard seeds

✓ 1/2 teaspoon turmeric powder

✓ 1/2 teaspoon ground coriander

✓ 1/2 teaspoon ground cumin

✓ 4 cups water

✓ 1/2 teaspoon salt (adjust to taste)

✓ Fresh cilantro leaves for garnish (optional)

✓ Lemon wedges for serving (optional)

Preparation:

1. Rinse 1/2 cup yellow mung dal and 1/2 cup basmati rice together under cold water until the water runs clear.

2. In a medium-sized pot, heat 1 tablespoon of ghee over medium heat.

3. Add 1 teaspoon cumin seeds and 1/2 teaspoon mustard seeds to the heated ghee. Allow them to sizzle.

4. Stir in 1/2 teaspoon turmeric powder, 1/2 teaspoon ground coriander, and 1/2 teaspoon ground cumin.

5. Sauté for 1-2 minutes until fragrant.

6. Add the rinsed yellow mung dal and basmati rice to the pot.

7. Stir to coat the grains with the spices.

8. Pour in 4 cups of water and add 1/2 teaspoon of salt. Stir well.

9. Bring the mixture to a boil, then reduce the heat to low, cover the pot, and simmer for 25-30 minutes or until the dal and rice are soft and well-cooked. Stir occasionally.

10. Garnish with fresh cilantro leaves if desired.

Total Nutritional Value (Approximate Per Serving): Calories: 328, Total Fat: 14.6g, Carbohydrates: 42.9g, Dietary Fiber: 7.2g, Sugars: 0.8g, Protein: 9.1g.

Preparation Time: 5 minutes

Cooking Time: 30 minutes

Serve the Kitchari Snack warm in small bowls. Optionally, squeeze fresh lemon juice over the top for added flavor. This Ayurvedic snack is not only delicious but also easy to digest and nourishing.

CHAPTER 7
HEALTHY DESSERTS FOR EACH DOSHA

1. Sweet Rice Pudding

Ingredients:

✓ 1/2 cup basmati rice

✓ 4 cups milk (dairy or plant-based)

✓ 1/2 cup jaggery or raw sugar

✓ 1/2 teaspoon cardamom powder

✓ 1/4 cup raisins

✓ 1/4 cup chopped almonds

✓ 1/4 cup chopped cashews

✓ 1 tablespoon ghee

✓ A pinch of saffron strands (optional)

✓ Chopped pistachios for garnish (optional)

Preparation:

1. Rinse 1/2 cup basmati rice under cold water until the water runs clear.

2. In a saucepan, combine the rinsed rice and 4 cups of milk. Bring to a boil, then reduce the heat to low, cover, and simmer for 20-25 minutes or until the rice is soft and the mixture thickens. Stir occasionally.

3. Add 1/2 cup of jaggery or raw sugar to the rice and milk mixture. Stir until the jaggery dissolves.

4. Stir in 1/2 teaspoon of cardamom powder for aromatic flavor.

5. In a separate pan, heat 1 tablespoon of ghee.

6. Add chopped almonds, cashews, and raisins.

7. Sauté until the nuts are golden and the raisins are plump.

8. Add this mixture to the rice pudding.

9. If using saffron, soak a pinch of saffron strands in a tablespoon of warm milk for a few minutes.

10. Add this saffron-infused milk to the rice pudding for a subtle fragrance and color.

11. Allow the rice pudding to cook for an additional 10-15 minutes on low heat until it reaches a creamy consistency. Stir occasionally to prevent sticking.

12. Garnish with chopped pistachios for a delightful crunch.

Total Nutritional Value (Approximate Per Serving): Calories: 700-800 (varies based on milk type), Total Fat: 25-30g (varies based on milk type and nut choice), Cholesterol: Varies based on milk type, Sodium: Varies, Total Carbohydrates: 120-130g (varies based on rice and sugar), Dietary Fiber: 1-2g, Sugars: 80-90g, Protein: 10-15g (varies based on milk type and nut choice).

Preparation Time: 5 minutes

Cooking Time: 45 minute

Serve the Sweet Rice Pudding warm or chilled, and savor the rich, comforting flavors of this Ayurvedic dessert. Enjoy it as a wholesome snack or a sweet treat after a meal.

2. Almond Halva

Ingredients:

✓ 1 cup almond flour

✓ 1/2 cup ghee

- ✓ 1/2 cup jaggery or raw sugar
- ✓ 1/4 cup water
- ✓ 1/2 teaspoon cardamom powder
- ✓ Chopped almonds for garnish (optional)

Preparation:

1. In a saucepan, combine 1/2 cup jaggery or raw sugar with 1/4 cup water. Heat over low heat, stirring until the jaggery dissolves.

2. If necessary, strain the syrup to eliminate contaminants.

3. In a separate pan, heat 1/2 cup of ghee over medium heat.

4. Add 1 cup of almond flour to the heated ghee.

5. Stir continuously to prevent lumps and ensure even roasting.

6. Continue roasting the almond flour in ghee until it turns golden brown and releases a nutty aroma.

7. This may take approximately 10-15 minutes.

8. Once the almond flour is well-roasted, slowly add the prepared jaggery syrup to the pan.

9. Keep stirring to combine the syrup with the almond flour.

10. Cook the mixture over low heat, stirring consistently until it thickens and reaches a halva-like consistency.

11. This usually takes about 10-15 minutes.

12. Stir in 1/2 teaspoon of cardamom powder for aromatic flavor.

13. Garnish the almond halva with chopped almonds for added texture.

Total Nutritional Value (Approximate Per Serving): Calories: 1983, Total Fat: 168g, Carbohydrates: 122g, Dietary Fiber: 12g, Sugars: 100g, Protein: 24.1g.

Preparation Time: 15 minutes

Cooking Time: 25-30 minutes

Serve the Almond Halva warm or at room temperature as a delicious and indulgent Ayurvedic snack. Enjoy the rich, nutty flavors and the sweetness of jaggery in this wholesome treat.

3. Carrot Halva

Ingredients:

✓ 2 cups grated carrots

✓ 1/2 cup ghee

✓ 1 cup milk (dairy or plant-based)

✓ 1/2 cup jaggery or raw sugar

✓ 1/2 teaspoon cardamom powder

✓ Garnish with chopped nuts (almonds, cashews, or pistachios).

✓ A pinch of saffron strands (optional)

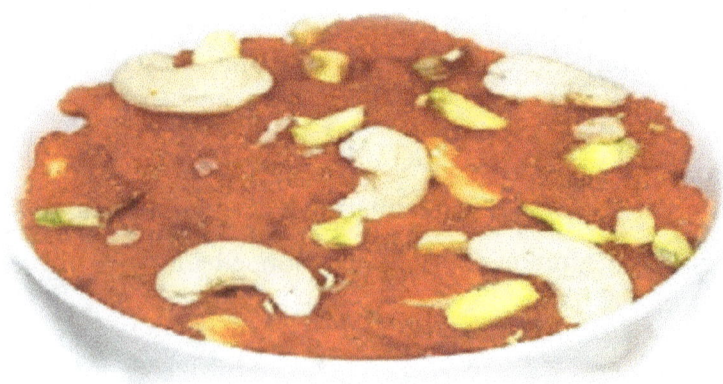

Preparation:

1. Grate 2 cups of carrots using a fine grater.

2. In a pan, heat 1/2 cup of ghee.

3. Add the grated carrots and sauté them until they become soft and release their aroma.

4. This may take around 10-15 minutes.

5. Pour in 1 cup of milk (dairy or plant-based) and continue cooking the carrots until the milk is absorbed and the mixture thickens. Stir occasionally.

6. Add 1/2 cup of jaggery or raw sugar to the pan.

7. Mix well and allow the jaggery to melt, creating a sweet syrup with the carrots.

8. Continue cooking the mixture on low heat until it reaches a halva-like consistency.

9. This may take approximately 15-20 minutes. Stir frequently to avoid sticking.

10. Stir in 1/2 teaspoon of cardamom powder for aromatic flavor.

11. Garnish the carrot halva with chopped nuts (almonds, cashews, or pistachios) for added crunch.

12. Add saffron strands for a hint of fragrance and color, if desired.

Total Nutritional Value (Approximate Per Serving): Calories: 1623-1663 (varies based on milk type), Total Fat: 116.4g, Carbohydrates: 129-135g (varies based on milk type and jaggery), Dietary Fiber: 7g, Sugars: 118g, Protein: 10.1g.

Preparation Time: 15 minutes

Cooking Time: 45-50 minutes

Serve the Carrot Halva warm or at room temperature, savoring the delightful blend of sweet carrots, rich ghee, and aromatic cardamom. This Ayurvedic snack makes for a satisfying and nourishing treat.

4. Coconut Ladoo

Ingredients:

✓ 2 cups desiccated coconut

✓ 1 cup condensed milk (sweetened)

✓ 1/2 cup ghee

✓ 1/2 teaspoon cardamom powder

✓ Garnish with chopped nuts (almonds, cashews, or pistachios).

Preparation:

1. In a pan, heat 1/2 cup of ghee. Add 2 cups of desiccated coconut and roast it on low heat until it turns golden brown. Stir continuously to avoid burning.

2. Once the coconut is roasted, pour in 1 cup of sweetened condensed milk.

3. To blend with the coconut, mix thoroughly.

4. Cook the mixture on low heat, stirring continuously, until it thickens and starts leaving the sides of the pan.

5. This may take around 10-15 minutes.

6. Stir in 1/2 teaspoon of cardamom powder for aromatic flavor.

7. Continue cooking until the mixture reaches a consistency suitable for shaping into ladoos.

8. Allow the mixture to cool slightly.

9. Ghee your hands and form the mixture into tiny, round ladoos.

10. Garnish the Coconut Ladoos with chopped nuts (almonds, cashews, or pistachios) for added texture.

Total Nutritional Value (Approximate Per Serving): Calories: 2900, Total Fat: 220g, Carbohydrates: 216g, Dietary Fiber: 32g, Sugars: 184g, Protein: 36g

Preparation Time: 10 minutes

Cooking Time: 20-25 minutes

Serve these delightful Coconut Ladoos as a sweet and nutritious Ayurvedic snack. Enjoy the rich coconut flavor and the goodness of condensed milk in every bite.

5. Cardamom Pistachio Ice Cream

Ingredients:

✓ 2 cups heavy cream

✓ 1 cup whole milk

✓ 3/4 cup granulated sugar

✓ 1 teaspoon ground cardamom

✓ 1/2 cup shelled pistachios, chopped

✓ 1 teaspoon vanilla extract

Preparation:

1. In a mixing bowl, combine 2 cups heavy cream, 1 cup whole milk, and 3/4 cup granulated sugar.

2. Add the sugar and whisk until it has dissolved.

3. Add 1 teaspoon ground cardamom to the cream mixture.

4. Whisk thoroughly to infuse the cardamom flavor.

5. Cover the bowl and refrigerate the mixture for at least 4 hours or overnight to allow the flavors to meld.

6. In a pan, lightly toast 1/2 cup chopped pistachios until they release their aroma. Allow them to cool.

7. Pour the cooled liquid into an ice cream machine and spin according to the manufacturer's guidelines.

8. During the last few minutes of churning, add the toasted pistachios and continue until well distributed.

9. Add 1 teaspoon of vanilla extract to the churned ice cream and mix until incorporated.

10. Transfer the ice cream to a covered container and freeze for at least 4-6 hours, or until hard.

Total Nutritional Value (Approximate Per Serving): Calories: 2540, Total Fat: 210g, Carbohydrates: 156g, Protein: 28g.

Preparation Time: 10 minutes

Chilling Time: 4 hours or overnight

Churning Time: According to ice cream maker instructions

Freezing Time: 4-6 hours

Scoop out the Cardamom Pistachio Ice Cream and enjoy the delightful combination of cardamom-spiced creaminess with the crunch of pistachios.

6. Mango Lassi

Ingredients:

✓ 1 cup ripe mango, peeled and diced

✓ 1 cup yogurt (preferably plain or Greek)

✓ 1/2 cup cold milk

✓ 2 tablespoons honey or sweetener of choice

✓ 1/2 teaspoon ground cardamom (optional)

✓ Ice cubes (optional)

✓ Fresh mint leaves for garnish (optional)

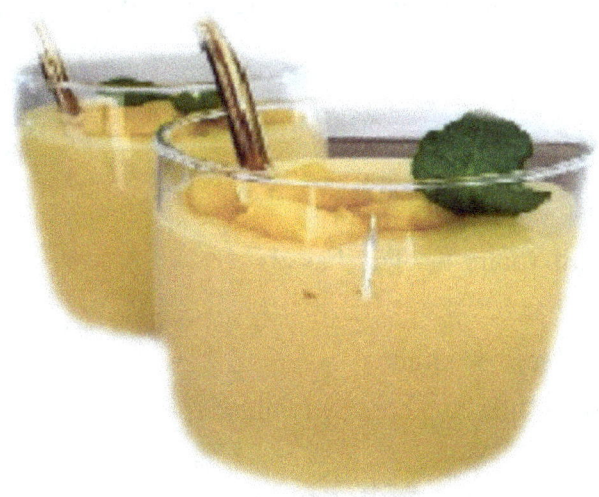

Preparation:

1. Peel and dice 1 cup of ripe mango.

2. In a blender, combine the diced mango, 1 cup yogurt, 1/2 cup cold milk, 2 tablespoons honey, and 1/2 teaspoon ground cardamom (if using).

3. Blend the ingredients together until smooth and fully incorporated.

4. Add ice cubes if a colder and thicker consistency is desired.

5. Taste the lassi and adjust sweetness by adding more honey if needed. Blend again to incorporate.

Total Nutritional Value (Approximate Per Serving): Calories: 400, Total Fat: 10.1g, Carbohydrates: 74.5g, Dietary Fiber: 3g, Sugars: 58g, Protein: 10.9g.

Preparation Time: 10 minutes

Pour the Mango Lassi into glasses, garnish with fresh mint leaves if desired, and enjoy this refreshing and nourishing Ayurvedic snack.

7. Saffron Rice Pudding

Ingredients:

✓ 1 cup basmati rice

✓ 4 cups milk (dairy or plant-based)

✓ 1/2 cup sugar

✓ A pinch of saffron strands

✓ 1/4 cup of finely chopped nuts (pistachios, cashews, or almonds)

✓ 1/2 teaspoon ground cardamom

✓ 1 teaspoon ghee (optional)

✓ Raisins for garnish (optional)

Preparation:

1. Use cold water to rinse one cup of basmati rice until the water runs clean.

2. In a saucepan, combine the rinsed rice and 4 cups of milk.

3. Cook over medium heat until the rice is soft and the mixture thickens, stirring occasionally.

4. While the rice is cooking, dissolve a pinch of saffron strands in a tablespoon of warm milk.

5. Add this saffron-infused milk to the rice and continue cooking.

6. Once the rice is nearly cooked, add 1/2 cup of sugar and stir until well combined. Adjust sweetness to taste.

7. Stir in 1/4 cup of chopped nuts (almonds, cashews, or pistachios) and continue cooking until the nuts are well incorporated.

8. Add 1/2 teaspoon of ground cardamom for a fragrant flavor. Mix well.

9. For added richness, stir in 1 teaspoon of ghee (clarified butter) if desired.

Total Nutritional Value (ApproximatePer Serving): Calories: 1600-1800 (varies based on milk type and nut choice), Total Fat: 50.5-64.5g (varies based on milk type and nut choice), Carbohydrates: 201-229g (varies based on milk type and nut choice), Dietary Fiber: 1, Protein: 42.3-46.3g (varies based on milk type and nut choice).

Preparation Time: 5 minutes

Cooking Time: 30-40 minutes

Garnish the Saffron Rice Pudding with raisins if desired. Serve warm or chilled for a delightful Ayurvedic snack or dessert.

8. Sweet Potato Pie

Ingredients:

For the Crust:

✓ 1 1/2 cups graham cracker crumbs

✓ 1/3 cup melted ghee or butter

✓ 1/4 cup sugar (optional)

For the Filling:

✓ 2 cups mashed sweet potatoes (equivalent to 2 medium sweet potatoes)

✓ 1/2 cup coconut sugar or brown sugar

✓ 1/2 cup of coconut milk (or any other plant-based milk)

✓ 2 large eggs

✓ 1 teaspoon vanilla extract

✓ 1/2 teaspoon ground cinnamon

✓ 1/4 teaspoon ground nutmeg

✓ A pinch of salt

For Topping (Optional):

✓ Whipped coconut cream or yogurt

✓ Chopped nuts (pecans or walnuts)

Preparation:

1. Preheat your oven to 350°F (175°C).

2. In a bowl, combine 1 1/2 cups graham cracker crumbs, 1/3 cup melted ghee or butter, and 1/4 cup sugar (optional). Mix until the crumbs are coated.

3. Press the mixture into the bottom and sides of a pie dish to form the crust.

4. Bake the crust for 8-10 minutes, or until it has set, in a preheated oven.

5. Remove from the oven and leave aside to cool.

6. Peel, dice, and boil 2 medium-sized sweet potatoes until they are soft.

7. Mash the sweet potatoes until smooth.

8. In a large bowl, combine 2 cups mashed sweet potatoes, 1/2 cup coconut sugar or brown sugar, 1/2 cup coconut milk or any plant-based milk, 2 large eggs, 1 teaspoon vanilla extract, 1/2 teaspoon ground cinnamon, 1/4 teaspoon ground nutmeg, and a pinch of salt. Mix until well combined.

9. Pour the sweet potato mixture into the baked crust. Smooth the top with a spatula.

10. Bake the sweet potato pie in the preheated oven for 45-50 minutes or until the center is set.

11. A toothpick put into the middle should come out clean.

12. Allow the pie to cool completely before transferring it to the refrigerator to chill for at least 2 hours or overnight.

Total Nutritional Value (Approximate Per Serving): Calories: 1850, Total Fat: 50.2g, Carbohydrates: 232g, Dietary Fiber: 8g, Sugars: 16g, Protein: 23g.

Preparation Time: 20 minutes

Baking Time: 45-50 minutes

Chilling Time: 2 hours or overnight

Serve the Sweet Potato Pie chilled, optionally topped with whipped coconut cream or yogurt and chopped nuts for added texture and flavor. Enjoy this Ayurvedic twist on a classic dessert!

9. Spiced Apple Crisp

Ingredients:

For the Filling:

✓ 6 cups thinly sliced apples (about 6 medium-sized apples, like Granny Smith or Honeycrisp)

✓ 1 tablespoon lemon juice

✓ 1/4 cup coconut sugar or brown sugar

✓ 1 teaspoon ground cinnamon

✓ 1/4 teaspoon ground nutmeg

✓ 1/4 teaspoon ground ginger

✓ 1/4 teaspoon salt

For the Topping:

✓ 1 cup old-fashioned rolled oats

✓ 1/2 cup almond flour

✓ 1/4 cup coconut sugar or brown sugar

✓ 1/4 cup melted ghee or coconut oil

✓ 1/2 teaspoon ground cinnamon

✓ 1/4 teaspoon salt

Preparation:

1. Preheat your oven to 350°F (175°C).

2. Peel, core, and thinly slice 6 medium-sized apples.

3. Mix the apple pieces with 1 tablespoon of lemon juice.

4. In a bowl, combine the sliced apples, 1/4 cup coconut sugar or brown sugar, 1 teaspoon ground cinnamon, 1/4 teaspoon ground nutmeg, 1/4 teaspoon ground ginger, and 1/4 teaspoon salt.

5. Mix until the apples are well coated.

6. Transfer the spiced apple mixture to a greased baking dish, spreading it evenly.

7. In another bowl, combine 1 cup old-fashioned rolled oats, 1/2 cup almond flour, 1/4 cup coconut sugar or brown sugar, 1/4 cup melted ghee or coconut oil, 1/2 teaspoon ground cinnamon, and 1/4 teaspoon salt.

8. Mix until it forms a crumbly texture.

9. Sprinkle the oat and almond topping evenly over the spiced apples in the baking dish.

10. Bake for 40-45 minutes, or until the topping is golden brown and the apples are soft, in a preheated oven.

Total Nutritional Value (Approximate Per Serving): Calories: 1830, Total Fat: 85.2g, Carbohydrates: 262g, Dietary Fiber: 29g, Sugars: 76g, Protein: 24g.

Preparation Time: 20 minutes

Baking Time: 40-45 minutes

Serve the Spiced Apple Crisp warm on its own or with a dollop of Greek yogurt or a scoop of vanilla ice cream for a delicious Ayurvedic snack or dessert. Enjoy the comforting flavors of spiced apples and a crunchy topping.

10. Date and Nut Balls

Ingredients:

- ✓ 1 cup of pitted Medjool dates (approximately 12-14 dates)
- ✓ 1 cup mixed nuts (almonds, walnuts, cashews), finely chopped
- ✓ 1/4 cup desiccated coconut
- ✓ 1 tablespoon chia seeds
- ✓ 1 tablespoon of nut butter, such as almond butter
- ✓ 1 teaspoon ground cinnamon
- ✓ A pinch of salt
- ✓ Additional desiccated coconut for coating (optional)

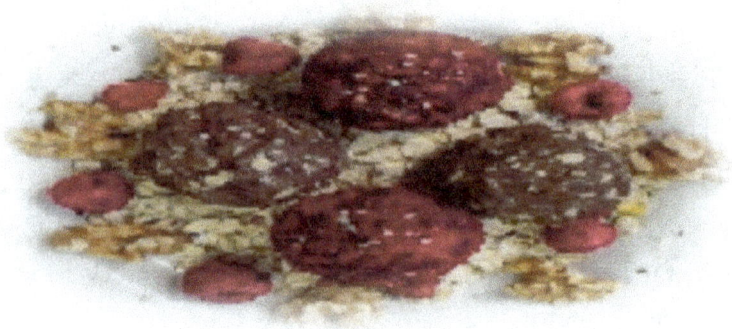

Preparation:

1. Remove pits from Medjool dates and chop them into smaller pieces.

2. In a dry skillet over medium heat, toast the mixed nuts until they become fragrant.

3. Be careful not to burn them.

4. Let them cool, then finely chop.

5. In a food processor, combine chopped dates, chopped nuts, desiccated coconut, chia seeds, almond butter, ground cinnamon, and a pinch of salt. Blend until the mixture forms a sticky dough.

6. Take small amounts of the mixture and roll them between your palms to make bite-sized balls.

7. If desired, roll the balls in additional desiccated coconut for a coating.

8. Place the date and nut balls in the refrigerator for at least 30 minutes to firm up.

Total Nutritional Value (Per Serving - Makes approximately 12 balls): Calories: 1248, Total Fat: 100.2g, Carbohydrates: 72g, Dietary Fiber: 25.5g, Sugars: 32g, Protein: 30.4g

Preparation Time: 15 minutess

Refrigeration Time: 30 minutes

Enjoy these Date and Nut Balls as a healthy and energizing Ayurvedic snack. They are perfect for satisfying sweet cravings while providing a nutrient-rich boost.

11. Coconut and Almond Fudge

Ingredients:

✓ 1 cup coconut butter

✓ 1/2 cup almond butter

✓ 1/4 cup raw honey or maple syrup

✓ 1/2 cup shredded coconut (unsweetened)

✓ 1/2 cup chopped almonds

✓ 1 teaspoon vanilla extract

✓ A pinch of salt

Preparation:

1. If your coconut butter is solid, gently heat it until it becomes soft and easy to mix.

2. In a mixing bowl, combine coconut butter, almond butter, raw honey or maple syrup, shredded coconut, chopped almonds, vanilla extract, and a pinch of salt.

3. Mix all ingredients thoroughly until you have a uniform and well-combined mixture.

4. Line a small tray or dish with parchment paper. Transfer the mixture to the tray and press it down evenly to form a solid layer.

5. Place the tray in the refrigerator and let it chill for at least 2-3 hours, or until the fudge is firm.

6. Once the fudge is set, remove it from the refrigerator and cut it into small squares or bars.

Total Nutritional Value (Per Serving - Makes approximately 12 squares): Calories: 2776, Total Fat: 259g, Carbohydrates: 137g, Dietary Fiber: 39g, Sugars: 92g, Protein: 47.3g.

Preparation Time: 15 minutes

Refrigeration Time: 2-3 hours

Enjoy this delicious Coconut and Almond Fudge as a satisfying Ayurvedic snack or dessert. The combination of coconut and almonds provides a delightful texture and flavor, making it a wholesome treat.

CHAPTER 8

BUILDING A 14 DAY BALANCED MEALS FOR YOUR DOSHA

Day 1

✓ *Breakfast:* Golden Milk Smoothie

Ingredients: Almond milk, turmeric, ginger, banana, honey

Nutritional Value: Rich in antioxidants, anti-inflammatory

✓ *Lunch:* Quinoa Salad with Tangy Tahini Sauce

Ingredients: Quinoa, mixed vegetables, chickpeas, tahini dressing

Nutritional Value: Protein, fiber, healthy fats

✓ *Dinner:* Healing Soup for Acid Reflux

Ingredients: Mung beans, basmati rice, digestive spices

Nutritional Value: Easy to digest, soothing for the digestive system

Day 2

✓ *Breakfast:* Fresh Homemade Yogurt with Berries

Ingredients: Yogurt, mixed berries, honey

Nutritional Value: Probiotics, antioxidants

✓ *Lunch:* Masala Rice (Vegetable Spiced Rice)

Ingredients: Brown rice, mixed vegetables, Indian spices

Nutritional Value: Fiber, complex carbohydrates, aromatic spices

✓ *Dinner:* Ayurvedic Kitchari with Cilantro and Coconut

Ingredients: Mung beans, basmati rice, coconut, cilantro

Nutritional Value: Balanced, easy to digest

Day 3

✓ *Breakfast:* Date-Plum Cream

Ingredients: Dates, plums, yogur

Nutritional Value: Natural sweetness, probiotics

✓ *Lunch:* Slow Cooker Quinoa Kichari

Ingredients: Quinoa, lentils, spices

Nutritional Value: Protein, fiber, one-pot convenience

✓ *Dinner:* Mediterranean Summer Salad

Ingredients: Mixed greens, olives, feta, olive oil dressing

Nutritional Value: Refreshing, light, Mediterranean flavors

Day 4

✓ *Breakfast:* Cream of Rice Soup (Congee)

Ingredients: Rice, vegetable broth, ginger, ghee

Nutritional Value: Comforting, easy to digest

✓ *Lunch:* Saffron Rice

Ingredients: Basmati rice, saffron, mixed vegetables

Nutritional Value: Aromatic, anti-inflammatory

✓ *Dinner:* Spiced Poha

Ingredients: Flattened rice, peas, mustard seeds, spice

Nutritional Value: Quick, flavorful, good for digestion

Day 5

✓ *Breakfast:* Sweet Rice Pudding

Ingredients: Basmati rice, milk, cardamom, nuts

Nutritional Value: Sweet, nourishing, traditional dessert

✓ *Lunch:* Clean Beets N Greens Kitchari

Ingredients: Mung beans, rice, beets, greens

Nutritional Value: Detoxifying, balancing

✓ *Dinner:* Masala Rice (Vegetable Spiced Rice)

Ingredients: Brown rice, mixed vegetables, Indian spices

Nutritional Value: Fiber, complex carbohydrates, aromatic spices

Day 6

✓ *Breakfast:* Frothy Almond Date Shake

Ingredients: Almond milk, dates, cinnamon

Nutritional Value: Energy-boosting, sweet, satisfying

✓ *Lunch:* Quinoa Salad with Tangy Tahini Sauce

Ingredients: Quinoa, mixed vegetables, chickpeas, tahini dressing

Nutritional Value: Protein, fiber, healthy fats

✓ **Dinner:** Ayurvedic Kitchari with Cilantro and Coconut

Ingredients: Mung beans, basmati rice, coconut, cilantro

Nutritional Value: Balanced, easy to digest

Day 7

✓ **Breakfast:** Golden Milk Smoothie

Ingredients: Almond milk, turmeric, ginger, banana, honey

Nutritional Value: Rich in antioxidants, anti-inflammatory

✓ *Lunch:* Healing Soup for Acid Reflux

Ingredients: Mung beans, basmati rice, digestive spices

Nutritional Value: Easy to digest, soothing for the digestive system

Dinner: Spiced Apple Crisp

Ingredients: Apples, cinnamon, oats, ghee

Nutritional Value: Warm dessert, comforting

Day 8

✓ **Breakfast:** Fresh Homemade Yogurt with Berries

Ingredients: Yogurt, mixed berries, honey

Nutritional Value: Probiotics, antioxidants

✓ *Lunch:* Slow Cooker Quinoa Kichari

Ingredients: Quinoa, lentils, spices

Nutritional Value: Protein, fiber, one-pot convenience

✓ *Dinner:* Sage Gravy with Roasted Vegetables

Ingredients: Ghee, whole wheat flour, sage, vegetables

Nutritional Value: Earthy, flavorful, comforting

Day 9

✓ *Breakfast:* Sweet Potato, Kale and Black Bean Bowl

Ingredients: Sweet potato, kale, black beans, spices

Nutritional Value: Satisfying, nutrient-rich

✓ *Lunch:* Mediterranean Summer Salad

Ingredients: Mixed greens, olives, feta, olive oil dressing

Nutritional Value: Refreshing, light, Mediterranean flavors

✓ *Dinner:* Masala Rice (Vegetable Spiced Rice)

Ingredients: Brown rice, mixed vegetables, Indian spices

Nutritional Value: Fiber, complex carbohydrates, aromatic spices

Day 10

✓ *Breakfast:* Date-Plum Cream

Ingredients: Dates, plums, yogurt

Nutritional Value: Natural sweetness, probiotics

✓ **Lunch:** Ayurvedic Kitchari with Cilantro and Coconut

Ingredients: Mung beans, basmati rice, coconut, cilantro

Nutritional Value: Balanced, easy to digest

✓ **Dinner:** Roasted Tandoori Cauliflower Bowls

Ingredients: Cauliflower, spices, quinoa

Nutritional Value: Spicy, flavorful, roasted goodness

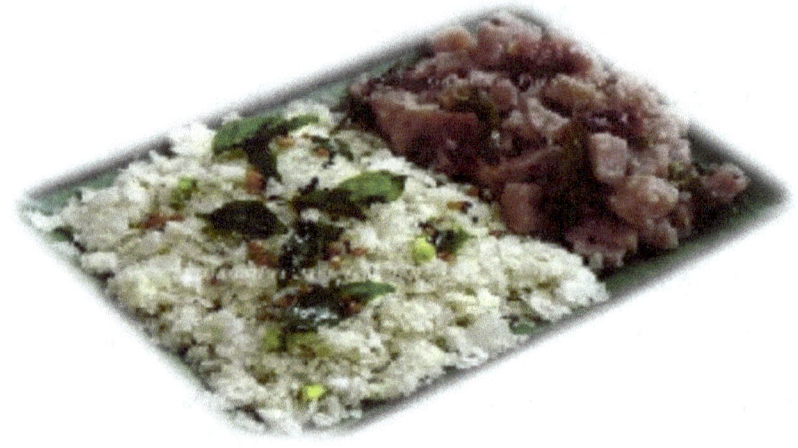

Day 11

✓ **Breakfast:** Golden Milk Smoothie

Ingredients: Almond milk, turmeric, ginger, banana, honey

Nutritional Value: Rich in antioxidants, anti-inflammatory

✓ **Lunch:** Spiced Poha

Ingredients: Flattened rice, peas, mustard seeds, spices

Nutritional Value: Quick, flavorful, good for digestion

✓ **Dinner:** Easy Indian-inspired Kitchari Bowls

Ingredients: Mung beans, rice, Indian spices, vegetables

Nutritional Value: Wholesome, comforting

Day 12

✓ **Breakfast:** Cream of Rice Soup (Congee)

Ingredients: Rice, vegetable broth, ginger, ghee

Nutritional Value: Comforting, easy to digest

✓ **Lunch:** Saffron Rice

Ingredients: Basmati rice, saffron, mixed vegetables

Nutritional Value: Aromatic, anti-inflammatory

✓ **Dinner:** Ayurvedic Kitchari with Cilantro and Coconut

Ingredients: Mung beans, basmati rice, coconut, cilantro

Nutritional Value: Balanced, easy to digest

Day 13

✓ **Breakfast:** Frothy Almond Date Shake

Ingredients: Almond milk, dates, cinnamon

Nutritional Value: Energy-boosting, sweet, satisfying

✓ **Lunch:** Quinoa Salad with Tangy Tahini Sauce

Ingredients: Quinoa, mixed vegetables, chickpeas, tahini dressing

Nutritional Value: Protein, fiber, healthy fats

✓ **Dinner:** Healing Soup for Acid Reflux

Ingredients: Mung beans, basmati rice, digestive spices

Nutritional Value: Easy to digest, soothing for the digestive system

Day 14

✓ **Breakfast:** Sweet Rice Pudding

Ingredients: Basmati rice, milk, cardamom, nuts

Nutritional Value: Sweet, nourishing, traditional dessert

✓ **Lunch:** Masala Rice (Vegetable Spiced Rice)

Ingredients: Brown rice, mixed vegetables, Indian spices

Nutritional Value: Fiber, complex carbohydrates, aromatic spices

✓ **Dinner:** Spiced Apple Crisp

Ingredients: Apples, cinnamon, oats, ghee

Nutritional Value: Warm dessert, comforting

Notes:

1. Adapt portion sizes based on individual needs

2. Hydration is essential; incorporate herbal teas and water throughout the day.

3. Listen to your body's appetite and fullness indicators.

This 14-day Ayurvedic meal plan incorporates a variety of flavors, textures, and nutrients, aligning with Ayurvedic principles to support balance and well-being.

CONCLUSION

As you close the pages of this Homemade Ayurveda Recipes cookbook, let the wisdom of this ancient healing system continue to guide you on your cooking journey. Remember, Ayurveda is not just about food; it's a holistic approach to living that encompasses mind, body, and spirit.

Embrace the principles of balance, harmony, and self-awareness that lie at the heart of Ayurveda. Listen to your body's cues, honor your unique constitution, and nourish yourself with wholesome, seasonal ingredients.

As you experiment with the recipes in this cookbook, you'll discover a world of flavors and a newfound appreciation for the transformative power of food. Let these recipes be the stepping stones on your path to a healthier, happier, and more fulfilling life.

Remember, Ayurveda is a journey, not a destination. Embrace the process, enjoy the exploration, and savor the nourishment that comes from cooking with love and intention.

I want to express my heartfelt gratitude for embarking on this culinary journey alongside me. Your willingness to explore the world of Ayurveda with an open mind and a curious palate is a testament to your commitment to your health and well-being.

I have poured my heart and soul into creating this cookbook, hoping to provide you with a valuable resource that goes beyond just recipes. My intention is to empower you with the knowledge and inspiration to integrate Ayurvedic principles into your daily life, transforming your relationship with food and embracing a lifestyle that nourishes your body and mind.

As you continue to explore the recipes and tips within these pages, remember that you are not alone in this journey. Millions of individuals around the world share similar experiences, and together, we can create a community of support and culinary inspiration.

Thank you for trusting me to guide you through this wonderful adventure. I am honored to have played a small role in your journey towards a healthier, happier you.

With gratitude and admiration.

Please email me at *loefflerlaura753@gmail.com* if you have any questions about Ayurveda or the recipes in this cookbook.

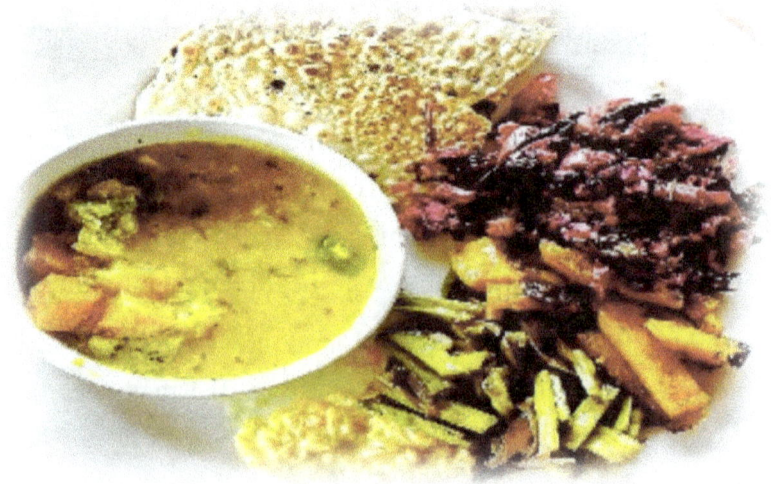

14 DAY MEAL PLANNER JOURNAL

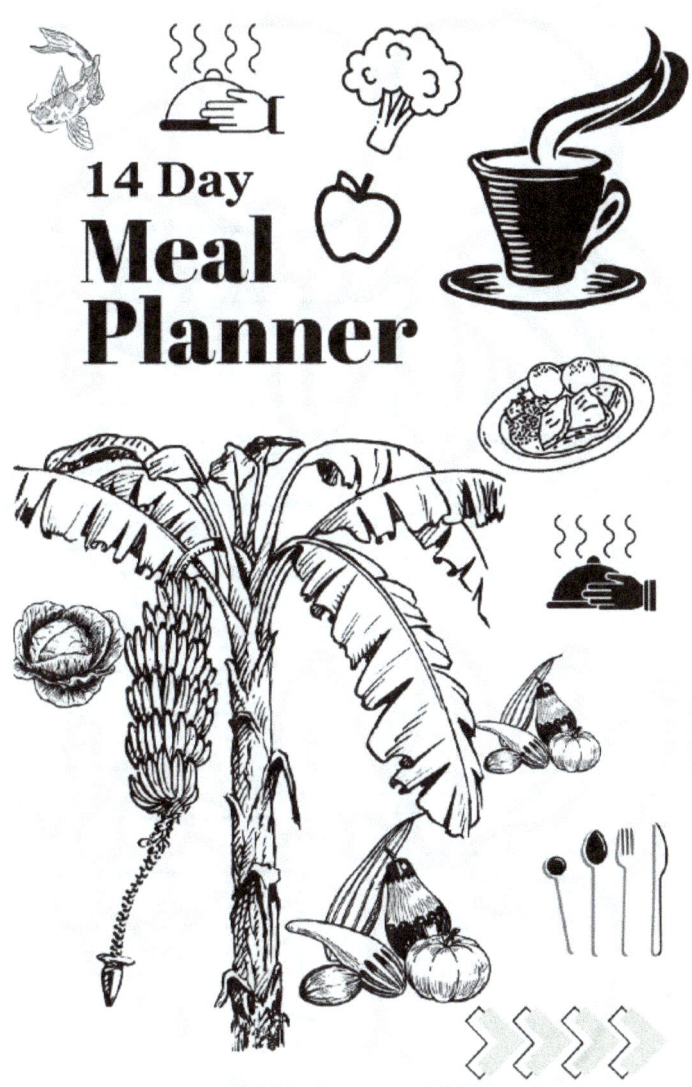

Date/Day: **Week:**

Water:

Menu List:

Breakfast:

Lunch:

Snacks:

Dinner:

Main Meal:

To Do List:

Shopping List:

☐ _____
☐ _____
☐ _____
☐ _____
☐ _____
☐ _____

TO BUY

SALAD

Note and Tips:

To-Do

Date/Day: **Week:**

Water:

Menu List:

Breakfast:

Lunch:

Snacks:

Dinner:

Main Meal:

To Do List:

Shopping List:

- [ ] _____
- [ ] _____
- [ ] _____
- [ ] _____
- [ ] _____
- [ ] _____

TO BUY

SALAD

Note and Tips:

To-Do

Date/Day: **Week:**

Water:

Menu List:

Breakfast:

Lunch:

Snacks:

Dinner:

Main Meal:

To Do List:

Shopping List:

☐ _____
☐ _____
☐ _____
☐ _____
☐ _____
☐

TO BUY

SALAD

Note and Tips:

To-Do

Date/Day: **Week:**   **Water:**

Menu List:

Breakfast:

Lunch:

Snacks:

Dinner:

Main Meal:

To Do List:

_____

_____

_____

_____

_____

Shopping List:

☐ _____
☐ _____
☐ _____
☐ _____
☐ _____
☐ _____

TO BUY

SALAD

Note and Tips:

To-Do

_____

_____

_____

_____

_____

_____

_____

Date/Day: **Week:**

Water:

Menu List:

Breakfast:

Lunch:

Snacks:

Dinner:

Main Meal:

To Do List:

Shopping List:

☐
☐
☐
☐
☐
☐

TO BUY

SALAD

Note and Tips:

To-Do

Date/Day: **Week:**

Water:

Menu List:

Breakfast:

Lunch:

Snacks:

Dinner:

Main Meal:

To Do List:

_____
_____
_____
_____
_____

Shopping List:

☐ _____
☐ _____
☐ _____
☐ _____
☐ _____
☐ _____

TO BUY

SALAD

Note and Tips:

★ **To-Do** ★

_____
_____
_____
_____
_____
_____

Date/Day: **Week:**

Water:

Menu List:

Breakfast:

Lunch:

Snacks:

Dinner:

Main Meal:

To Do List:

_____

_____

_____

_____

_____

Shopping List:

☐ _____
☐ _____
☐ _____
☐ _____
☐ _____
☐ _____

TO BUY

SALAD

Note and Tips:

To-Do

_____

_____

_____

_____

_____

_____

Date/Day: **Week:**

Water:

Menu List:

Breakfast:

Lunch:

Snacks:

Dinner:

Main Meal:

To Do List:

Shopping List:

TO BUY

SALAD

Note and Tips:

To-Do

Date/Day: **Week:**

Water:

Menu List:

Breakfast:

Lunch:

Snacks:

Dinner:

Main Meal:

To Do List:

Shopping List:

Note and Tips:

To-Do

Date/Day:　　　**Week:**　　　**Water:** ▮ ▮ ▮

Menu List:

Breakfast:

Lunch:

Snacks:

Dinner:

Main Meal:

To Do List:

_____

_____

_____

_____

_____

Shopping List:

☐ _____

☐ _____

☐ _____

☐ _____

☐ _____

☐ _____

TO BUY

Note and Tips:

★ To-Do ★

_____

_____

_____

_____

_____

_____

Date/Day: **Week:**

Water:

Menu List:

Breakfast:

Lunch:

Snacks:

Dinner:

Main Meal:

To Do List:

Shopping List:

☐ _____
☐ _____
☐ _____
☐ _____
☐ _____
☐ _____

TO BUY

SALAD

Note and Tips:

To-Do

Date/Day: **Week:**

Water:

Menu List:

Breakfast:

Lunch:

Snacks:

Dinner:

Main Meal:

To Do List:

Shopping List:

- [ ] _____
- [ ] _____
- [ ] _____
- [ ] _____
- [ ] _____
- [ ] _____

TO BUY

SALAD

Note and Tips:

To-Do

Date/Day: **Week:**

Water:

Menu List:

Breakfast:

Lunch:

Snacks:

Dinner:

Main Meal:

To Do List:

Shopping List:

- [ ] _____
- [ ] _____
- [ ] _____
- [ ] _____
- [ ] _____
- [ ] _____

TO BUY

SALAD

Note and Tips:

★ **To-Do** ★